MW00913144

THE PEDIATRIC

SURVIVAL GUIDE

Lisa M. Rebeschi, MSN, Doctoral Student, RN
Mary L. Brown, MSN, RN, LPNP

SKIDMORE-ROTH PUBLISHING, INC.

Cover design: Robert Pawlak

Typesetting: Affiliated Executive Systems

First edition

Notice: The author(s) and the publisher of this volume have taken care to make certain that all information is correct and compatible with the standards generally accepted at the time of publication.

Skidmore-Roth Publishing, Inc.
2020 S. Parker Road, Suite 147
Aurora, Colorado 80014
800-825-3150

TABLE OF CONTENTS

CLINICAL VALUES AND STANDARDS

DRUG ADMINISTRATION

CLINICAL SKILLS

DISEASE PROCESSES AND COMMON PROBLEMS

CLINICAL REFERRALS

INTRODUCTION

INTRODUCTION
TABLE OF CONTENTS

HOW TO USE THIS BOOK

The Pediatric Survival Guide is designed to accompany the Nurse's Survival Guide. The book should be used as a pediatric clinical practice reference guide. It was written by two nurse educators who are experts in pediatric nursing practice.

This book includes clinical information which pediatric nurses often use and it contains guidelines for care, formats for assessments, drug information, frequently practiced clinical skills, clinical values and standards, common disease processes/problems, caring for chronically ill children, dealing with dying, and many pediatric resources/referral agencies.

The book is not designed as a pediatric textbook, but as a quick reference. When additional information is needed, the nurse should consult a comprehensive pediatric text.

STANDARDS OF MATERNAL AND CHILD HEALTH NURSING PRACTICE

(developed by the American Nurses' Association, 1983)

STANDARD I: The nurse helps children and parents attain and maintain optimum health.

Rationale — "Attainment of optimum physical and psychological health by family members is the ultimate goal of health care. Nurses are in a unique position to help clients and/or families achieve this goal. Health-oriented nursing interventions include health teaching, anticipatory guidance, assistance in problem solving, and identification of actual or potential health problems and treatment and referral."

STANDARD II: The nurse assists families to achieve and maintain a balance between the personal growth needs of individual family members and optimum family functioning.

Rationale — "Families seek to provide for the physical, psychological, and cultural needs of their members. Nursing assists clients and families in the attainment of optimum family relationships and family functioning. In addition, nursing helps families achieve a balance that respects the personal growth needs of all family members by carrying out nursing interventions that enhance role development."

STANDARD III: The nurse intervenes with vulnerable clients and families at risk to prevent potential developmental and health problems.

Rationale — "Individuals and families at risk are particularly vulnerable to potential health problems. Nursing seeks to identify individuals and families at risk. It also monitors them and provides protective intervention either independently or collaboratively."

STANDARD IV: The nurse promotes an environment free of hazards to reproduction, growth and development, wellness, and recovery from illness.

Rationale — "Nurses have historically been concerned with the provision of an environment which promotes health. Hazards in the environment can jeopardize reproduction, growth and development, and health status. Nurses are often in a position to detect environmental hazards and help clients learn how to maintain a safe environment."

STANDARD V: The nurse detects changes in health status and deviations from optimum development.

Rationale — "Early detection of deviations in health and optimum development and changes in health status are essential to the prevention of illness. Nurses are in a unique position to detect these changes, initiate treatment, and promote development and health potential."

STANDARD VI: The nurse carries out appropriate interventions and treatment to facilitate survival and recovery from illness.

Rationale — "Acute care nursing requires assessment and diagnosis of the physiologic and psychological reactions of clients to illness and detection of changes in status. Nursing interventions in the independent practice domain are directed toward alleviation or resolution of problems such as pain, separation anxiety, self-care deficit, or alteration in body image. Nursing also provides a physical and psychological environment conducive to recovery and restoration of health. Nursing interventions in the interdependent practice domain, carried out in collaboration with physicians, are directed toward the alleviation or resolution of illness-related conditions."

STANDARD VII: The nurse assists clients and families to understand and cope with developmental and traumatic situations during illness, childbearing, childrearing, and childhood.

Rationale — "Clients of maternal and child health nurses often experience developmental and/or situational crises. Due to the closeness of their relationships with clients, nurses are in a unique position to practice crisis intervention. Nursing interventions are designed to help clients and families reduce or manage stress and facilitate adaptive coping."

STANDARD VIII: The nurse actively pursues strategies to enhance access to and utilization of adequate health care services.

Rationale — "The quality of health or childbearing and childrearing families depends on the availability and utilization of adequate health care services. MCH nursing assists clients to utilize appropriate health care services and resources. In addition, MCH nursing collaborates with consumers, other health disciplines, and governmental agencies in efforts to insure the availability and adequacy of health care services."

STANDARD IX: The nurse improves maternal and child health nursing practice through evaluation of practice, education, and research.

Rationale - "Improvement of the practice of maternal and child health nursing depends upon a commitment of the nurses in this field to participate in programs of practice evaluation, to acquire additional knowledge through informal and formal education, to use new knowledge and research findings in practice, to participate with others in research activities, to carry out own nursing research, and to disseminate research findings. Outcomes are measured in terms of behaviors of maternal and child health nurses."

THE MARK OF A PROFESSIONAL NURSE

The basic requirements of a profession are:

- Educational requirements;
- Unique knowledge and skills based upon theory;
- Service to society;
- Autonomy in decision-making and practice;
- A code of ethics for practice; and
- Some degree of status within the role.

These requirements are inherent in the foundation of professional nursing. The profession of compassionate caring that Florence Nightingale embraced for nursing is the interpersonal expertise unique to each nurse. These interpersonal skills are intimately intertwined with the professional skills.

Interpersonal skills encompass all the human actions that respect the body, mind and spirit of another person. It is looking at the patient with kindness, listening with empathy and responding with compassion. A professional nurse offers much more than technical skills, although more and more technical skills are required. It is the interpersonal skills that exhibit caring, confidentiality and positive regard for the patient in a holistic vision that are most valued in the professional nurse.

What do patients want in a nurse? This question was asked of several patients in the process of writing this book. What they want is empathy, sensitivity, experience (skills), caring and a sense of confidence, in that order. What they do not want is a nurse who is insensitive, in a hurry, with an air of power. Patients tend to feel very uncomfortable around nurses who seem unsure of what they are doing.

The quality of caring is not measured by time. The wink of an eye, the flash of a smile, the tenderness of a touch does not require extra time—it demonstrates nursing care.

It is impossible to label the characteristic that makes a nurse professional. That essential quality is elusive, perhaps indescribable. But, when you meet a nurse that has it, you know.

STANDARDS OF PROFESSIONAL PERFORMANCE

"Standards of Professional Performance" describe a competent level of behavior in the professional role including activities related to quality of care, performance appraisal, education, collegiality, ethics, collaboration, research, and resource utilization. All nurses are expected to engage in professional role activities appropriate to their education, position, and practice setting. While this is an assumption of all of the "Standards of Professional Performance", the scope of nursing involvement in some professional roles is particularly dependent upon the nurse's education, position, and practice environment. Therefore, some standards or measurement criteria identify a broad range of activities that may demonstrate compliance with the standards.

STANDARDS OF CARE

Standard I. Assessment

The Nurse collects Client Health Data.

Measurement Criteria

1. The priority of data collection is determined by the client's immediate condition or needs.

2. Pertinent data are collected using appropriate assessment techniques.

3. Data collection involves the client, significant others, and health care providers when appropriate.

4. The data collection process is systematic and ongoing.

5. Relevant data are documented in a retrievable form.

Standard II. Diagnosis

The nurse analyzes the assessment data in determining diagnoses.

Measurement Criteria

1. Diagnoses are derived from the assessment data.

2. Diagnoses are validated with the client, significant others, and health care providers, when possible.

3. Diagnoses are documented in a manner that facilitates the determination of unexpected outcomes and plan of care.

Standard III. Outcome Identification

The nurse identifies expected outcomes individualized to the client.

Measurement Criteria

1. Outcomes are derived from the diagnoses.

2. Outcomes are documented as measurable goals.

3. Outcomes are mutually formulated with the client and health care providers, when possible.

4. Outcomes are realistic in relation to the client's present and potential capabilities.

5. Outcomes are attainable in relation to resources available to the client.

6. Outcomes include a time estimate for attainment.

7. Outcomes provide direction for continuity of care.

Standard IV. Planning

The nurse develops a plan of care that prescribes interventions to attain expected outcomes.

Measurement Criteria

1. The plan is individualized to the client's condition or needs.

2. The plan is developed with the client, significant others, and health care providers, when appropriate.

3. The plan reflects current nursing practice.

4. The plan is documented.

5. The plan provides for continuity of care.

Standard V. Implementation

The nurse implements the interventions identified in the plan of care.

Measurement Criteria

1. Interventions are consistent with the established plan of care.

2. Interventions are implemented in a safe and appropriate manner.

3. Interventions are documented.

Standard VI. Evaluation

The nurse evaluates the client's progress toward attainment of outdoes.

Measurement Criteria

1. Evaluation is systematic and ongoing.

2. The client's responses to interventions are documented.

3. The effectiveness of interventions is evaluated in relation to outcomes.

4. Ongoing assessment data are used to revise diagnoses, outcomes, and the plan of care, as needed.

5. Revisions in diagnoses, outcomes, and the plan of care are documented

6. The client, significant others, and health care providers are involved in the evaluation process, when appropriate.

STANDARDS OF PROFESSIONAL PERFORMANCE

Standard I. Quality of Care

The nurse systematically evaluates the quality and effectiveness of nursing practice.

Measurement Criteria

1. The nurse participates in quality of care activities as appropriate to the individual's position, education, and practice environment. Such activities may include:
   - Identification of aspects of care important for quality monitoring.
   - Identification of indicators used to monitor quality and effectiveness of nursing care.
   - Collection of data to monitor quality and effectiveness of nursing care.
   - Analysis of quality data to identify opportunities for improving care.

- Formulation of recommendations to improve nursing practice or client outcomes.
- Implementation of activities to enhance the quality of nursing practice.
- Participation on interdisciplinary teams that evaluate clinical practice or health services.
- Development of policies and procedures to improve quality of care.

2. The nurse uses the results of quality of care activities to initiate changes in practice.
3. The nurse uses the results of quality of care activities to initiate changes throughout the health care delivery system, as appropriate.

Standard II. Performance Appraisal

The nurse evaluates his/her own nursing practice in relation to professional practice standards and relevant statutes and regulations.

Measurement Criteria

1. The nurse engages in performance appraisal on a regular basis, identifying areas of strength as well as areas for professional/practice development.
2. The nurse seeks constructive feedback regarding his/her own practice.
3. The nurse takes action to achieve goals identified during performance appraisal.
4. The nurse participates in peer review as appropriate.

Standard III. Education

The nurse acquires and maintains current knowledge in nursing practice.

Measurement Criteria

1. The nurse participates in ongoing educational activities related to clinical knowledge and professional issues.

2. The nurse seeks experiences to maintain clinical skills.

3. The nurse seeks knowledge and skill appropriate to the practice setting.

Standard IV. Collegiality

The nurse contributes to the professional development of peers, colleagues, and others.

Measurement Criteria

1. The nurse shares knowledge and skill with colleagues and others.

2. The nurse provides peers with constructive feedback regarding their practice.

3. The nurse contributes to an environment that is conducive to clinical education of nursing students, as appropriate.

Standard V. Ethics

The nurse's decisions and actions on behalf of clients are determined in an ethical manner.

Measurement Criteria

1. The nurse's practice is guided by the Code for Nurses.

2. The nurse maintains client confidentiality.

3. The nurse acts as a client advocate.

4. The nurse delivers care in a nonjudgmental and nondiscriminatory manner that is sensitive to client diversity.

5. The nurse delivers in a manner that preserves/protects client autonomy, dignity, and rights.

6.   The nurse seeks available resources to help formulate
     ethical decisions.

Standard VI. Collaboration

The nurse collaborates with the client, significant others, and
health care providers in providing client care.

Measurement Criteria

1.   The nurse communicates with the client, significant others,
     and health care providers regarding client care and
     nursing's role in the provision of care.

2.   The nurse consults with health care providers for client
     care, as needed.

3.   The nurse makes referrals, including provisions for
     continuity of care, as needed.

Standard VII. Research

The nurse uses research findings in practice.

Measurement Criteria

1.   The nurse uses interventions substantiated by research as
     appropriate to the individual's position, education, and
     practice environment.

2.   The nurse participates in research activities as appropriate
     to the individual's position, education, and practice
     environment. Such activities may include:
     • Identification of clinical problems suitable for nursing
       research.
     • Participation in data collection.
     • Participation in a unit, organization, or community
       research committee or program.
     • Sharing of research activities with others.
     • Conducting research.
     • Critiquing research for application to practice.

- Using research findings in the development of policies, procedures, and guidelines for client care.

Standard VIII. Resource Utilization

The nurse considers factors related to safety, effectiveness, and cost in planning and delivering client care.

Measurement Criteria.

1. The nurse evaluates factors related to safety effectiveness, and cost when two or more practice options would result in the same expected client outcome.

2. The nurse assigns tasks or delegates care based on the needs of the client and the knowledge and skill of the provider selected.

3. The nurse assists the client and significant others in identifying and securing appropriate services available to address health-related needs.

Printed with permission of the American Nurses Association from the ANA's Standards of Nursing Practice, 1991.

ASSESSMENT

COMMUNICATION WITH CHILDREN/FAMILIES

Basic Principles

—Privacy is an essential component.
—Be sure to properly identify yourself, your role, and purpose.
—Assure confidentiality.
—Begin communication with general content before getting specific.
—Communicate directly with child even when accompanied by adult.
—Remember that adolescents may need to communicate in private without the presence of family members.
—Use open ended questions.
—Encourage continued communication by nodding and eye contact.
—Recognize and be respectful of cultural influences on communication.
—Use silence when necessary.
—Active listening to both nonverbal and verbal cues is critical.
—Ensure mutual understanding.
—Avoid communication blocks (i.e., deliberate changing of focus, false reassurance, interrupting, close ended questions.
—Maintain eye level position with child.
—Transition objects such as stuffed animals may be useful to communicate through.
—Honesty is of ultimate importance.

PHYSICAL ASSESSMENT

GENERAL GUIDELINES

Be prepared with all equipment when you enter room. Take the stethoscope, tape measure, pen light, tongue blade, etc.

Establish rapport with parent and child by talking first. Use play therapy as necessary to accomplish assessment. Have child listen to mom's or bear's heart, lungs, to show child, especially toddler, that it doesn't hurt. Begin assessing as soon as you enter the room. Note skin color, position, gait if running away from you, parent response, and parent-child interaction. Complete assessment as opportunity presents. If an infant is sleeping, listen to heart sounds. If crying, breath sounds can be adequate. Save invasive procedures until the end; these vary with age groups. Ears, mouths, noses are invasive to a toddler. GU and abdomen are invasive to a schoolager or adolescent. Also, save painful areas until last. Allow the child to assist as able. Preschoolers and older children like to listen to their own heart sounds and you can utilize assessment as a teaching opportunity to teach the child about their body and how to keep it healthy and to validate normalcy. Regardless of what order in which assessment was done, it must be charted in logical head to toe format.

General Appearance
Note overall impression, state of consciousness. Ex: small, obese, well-nourished, awake, alert, cooperative, age or developmentally appropriate, lethargic.

Skin
Inspect and palpate for color (remember room color, gown color and lighting affect observation, evaluate for jaundice in natural lighting of the window, cyanosis blanches momentarily, bruises do not.) pigmentation, temperature, texture, moisture, and turgor. Note and describe all lesions for:

Location—exactly where on body

Pattern—clustered, confluent, evanescent
Size—measure in cm.
Color—red, pink, brown, white
Elevation—raised(papular),   flat(macular),   fluid   filled
    (vesicular)
Blanching—do they blanch with pressure.

Hair
Note color, texture, distribution, quality, and loss. Look in hair behind the ears for nits.

Nails
Note color, cyanosis, shape, condition, and for clubbing by checking nail angle. Normal angle is 160 degrees. 180 degree angle and larger is seen in clubbing due to hypoxia.

Head
Inspect and palpate. Feel for bogginess, palpate sutures, fontanelles. osterior fontanelle normally closes from birth to 2 months. Usually 1-2cm in size. Anterior fontanelle normally closes between 9-18 months but should be closed by 2 years. Measure anterior fontanelle in two dimensions. Usually is 4-5cm by 3-4cm, but should be at least 1cm by 1cm. Measure FOC until 2 years old or if its size is important to child's condition after 2 years. Always plot FOC. Note size, shape, and symmetry of head. Palpate scalp for tenderness and lesions.

Neck
Inspect for swelling, webbing, nuchal fold, vein distention. Palpate for swelling, carotid pulse, trachea, and thyroid.

Ears
Inspect for shape, color, symmetry, helix formation, position.
Top of ear should go through an imaginary line from the inner to thc outer canthus to the occiput.
Palpate for firmness and pain. Observe for and describe any discharge from ear canal.

Assess for gross hearing. Infants less than 4 months will startle to sound. Older infants will turn to localize the sound of jingling keys, etc. Use whisper test with verbal and cooperative children.

Eyes
Inspect for position, alignment, lid closure, inner canthal distance (Ave. 2.5 cm), for epicanthal folds, slant of fissure.
Brows—note separateness, nits.
Lashes—note if curve into eye itself
Lids—note color, swelling, lesions, discharge
Conjunctiva(Palpebral)—should be pink. Note redness, paleness, and pallor.
Sclera and bulbar conjunctiva—note injection, redness, color (Yellow in jaundice, blue in osteogenesis imperfecta).
Pupils—should be round, react briskly to light by constricting directly and consensually and accommodate for near and far vision.
Iris—note color, roundness, any clefts or defects.
EOM's (Extraocular Movements)
    Corneal light reflex—light held 15 inches from bridge of nose should reflect in same place in normally aligned eye.
    Cover-uncover test—check for movement when one eye is covered and the other is gazing at a distant object. Remove cover and note movement of covered eye.
    Six Cardinal Fields of Gaze—move your finger in shape of an H. Hold child's chin and have him follow your finger with his eyes to note asymmetric eye movement or to elicit nystagmus. A few beats of nystagmus in the far lateral gaze is normal.
Gross Vision—Infants who can see will fix on and follow objects. Can grossly assess older child's vision by having them describe what they see on the wall or out the window.

Face
Note color, symmetrical movement, expression, skin folds, swelling.

Nose
Note color of skin, nasal mucosa, any discharge and its color, and for patency. Remember, infants are obligate nose breathers until around 3 months of age.
Palpate sinuses for tenderness.

Mouth
Inspect all areas. Note number and condition of teeth. To calculate expected number of teeth in infants, subtract 6 from the age in months. Ex.: 12 months minus 6 = 6 teeth.
Observe tonsils for swelling (grade 1+ to kissing tonsils being 4+), color (should be same color as buccal mucosa), and discharge.
Note hard and soft palate for color, patency, and lesions.
Note uvula, should raise symmetrically, a bifid uvual could indicate a submucosal cleft.
Note tongue shape, size, color, movement and for any lesions. (Most common lesions are white and are thrush.)
Note breath odor.

Thorax and Lungs
Inspect for symmetry, movement, color, retractions, breast development, and type and effort of breathing. Breathing is predominately abdominal until 7 years. Note nasal flaring and use of accessory muscles. Retractions usually start subcostal and substernal then progress to suprasternal and clavicular, and lastly intercostal indicating severe distress.
Palpate for tactile fremitus-is increased in congestion and consolidation.
Percuss for resonance. Sound becomes dull with fluid or masses.
Auscultate side to side for symmetry of sound. Infants breath deeper when they cry, toddlers and preschoolers can breathe deeper when they blow bubbles or try to "blow out the light" of your pen light. Assess all fields. Must listen to the back to get lower lobes in children under 8 years. Auscultate in the axilla to hear crackles best in children with pneumonia.

Normal sounds are vesicular or bronchovesicular. Infants breath sounds are louder and more bronchial sounding because of thin chest walls.

Describe adventitious sounds as:

> Rhonchi—continuous, low-pitched sound with a snoring quality.
>
> Crackles—intermittent, brief, repetitive sounds due to small collapsed airways popping open.
>
> Fine—soft, high-pitched and brief
>
> Coarse—louder, lower-pitched and slightly longer
>
> Wheezes—musical, more continuous sounds produced by rapid movement of air through narrowed passages.
>
> > Stages of Wheezes:
> >
> > +   (1) Expiratory wheezes only
> >
> > + +   (2) Inspiratory wheezes with decreased expiratory wheezes
> >
> > + + +   (3) Inspiratory wheezes only, airways are collapsing on expiration.
> >
> > + + + +   (4) No sounds, little air is moving
>
> Stridor—inspiratory wheeze heard louder in neck than chest

Infants with upper airway congestion, can have sounds transmitted to lungs because of being obligate nose breathers. Listen to their lungs when they are crying and breathing through their mouth to decrease the amount of transmitted noise and better assess their breath sounds.

Cardiovascular (CV)

Inspect for PMI (point of maximum impulse), cyanosis, mottling, edema, respiratory distress, clubbing, activity intolerance, and tiring with feeds.

Palpate PMI, brachial, radial, femoral, and pedal pulses.

Auscultate with bell and diaphragm:

> Aortic area   Right 2nd intercostal space(ICS) at right sternal border(SB)

Pulmonic area	Left 2nd ICS at left SB
Erb's Point	Left 3rd ICS at left SB
Tricuspid	Left 5th ICS at left SB
Mitral	Left 5th ICS at left midclavicular line(MCL)

S1 correlates with the carotid pulse and is best heard at the apex of the heart. S2 is best heard in the aortic and pulmonic areas (Base of heart). Note quality of sound. Should be crisp and clear. Rate should be normal for age and condition and synchronous with the radial pulse. Rhythm should be regular or may slow and speed up with respirations in young infants.

Auscultate with child in two positions if possible.

Auscultate for muffled or additional sounds and note where these are best heard.

Murmurs should be assessed for the following:

Location—Where heard best on the chest wall

Timing in cardiac cycle—continuous, systolic, or diastolic if possible.

Grade—I-VI/VI

I — very faint

II — quiet, but can hear soon after placing stethoscope

III — moderately loud

IV — loud

V — very loud, may be heard with stethoscope partially off chest

VI — can be heard without the stethoscope

Pitch—High (best heard with the diaphragm), medium, or low (best heard with the bell)

Quality—Harsh, blowing, machinery-like, musical

Radiation—does it radiate and if so, where. Listen to back axilla, and above clavicles.

Abdomen

Inspect for pulsations, contour, symmetry, peristaltic waves, masses, and normal skin color.

Auscultate before palpating so normal bowel sounds aren't disturbed. Listen in all four quadrants for a full minute. Should hear normal sounds every 10-30 seconds. Should hear 4-5/min. Less than 4/min. Would indicate decreased bowel sounds. Listen for a full 5 minutes before concluding that they are absent.

Percuss for dullness over liver and full bladder. Rest of abdomen should percuss tympani.

Palpate using light pressure first. Have child bend knees up while lying on their back to relax abdomen. May use child's hands under your hands if they are very ticklish or tense. With deep palpation, support from back then palpate. Start in lower quadrants and move upward to detect enlarged liver or spleen.

Note areas of tenderness, pain or any masses.

Anus
Inspect skin and perineum for excoriation, bruising, discoloration, or tears.

Genitourinary (GU)
Female genitalia—note redness, excoriation, discharge and odor.
Male genitalia—note if circumcised or uncircumcised. If uncircumcised, see if foreskin is retractable. Note position of meatus. Close off the canals and feel for the testes or any masses in the scrotal sac. If a mass is felt other than the teste, transilluminate for fluid. Hydroceles are fluid and will transilluminate light. Hernias are loops of bowel and will not transilluminate.

Lymphatic System
Palpate throughout exam with pads of fingers. Nodes should be firm, small (1 cm or less), freely moveable, and nontender.
Palpate preauricular, postauricular, anterior and posterior cervical chains, supra and sub clavicular, axillary, and inguinal.

Musculoskeletal System
Incorporate into rest of exam. Observe walking, sitting, turning, and range of motion in all joints. Observe spinal curvature, mobility.

Exaggerated lumbar curve is normal in toddlers. Note sacral dimples or tufts of hair at the base of the spinal column.
Note symmetry and movement of extremities.
Test muscle strength. Strength is graded on a 0-5 scale:

    0—no contraction noted
    1—barely a trace of contraction
    2—active movement without gravity
    3—active movement against gravity
    4—active movement against gravity and resistance
    5—active movement against full resistance without tiring
       5 is normal muscle strength

Note size, color, temperature, mobility of joints. Look at palmar creases. Single crease is a Simian crease and can be associated with Down syndrome. Note extra digits and deformities. Thumb deformities may be associated with heart defects. Note stance and gait. Bowed legs (Genu varum) are normal in toddlers until around age 2 years. Knock knees (Genu valgum) are normal from 2 until around 6-10 years. Note foot deformities. Stroke the side of foot to see if it returns to a neutral position. Check for dislocatable hips using the Barlow's and Ortolani's maneuvers. Also look for uneven skin folds.

Nervous System

Observe grossly for ability to follow directions and speech in a older child. In a infant, observe activity and tone.
In ambulatory patients can observe gait, balance.
Check deep tendon reflexes. Are graded 0-4+.

    4+   very brisk, hyperactive
    3+   brisker than average
    2+   normal
    1+   decreased
    0   absent

Can use a percussion hammer or the side of the stethoscope diaphragm to elicit.

Deep Tendon Reflex		**Response**
Biceps	Hit antecubital space	forearm flexes
Triceps	Bend arm at elbow, hit triceps tendon above the elbow	forearm extends
Patellar	Strike patellar tendon	lower leg extends
Achilles	hold foot lightly, hit achilles tendon	foot flexes downward

Cranial nerves—most are integrated into rest of exam and are not routinely tested.

Infant Reflexes

Reflex	**Timing**	**Assessment**
Babinski	Birth-2 yr.	Toes fan when bottom of foot is stroked
Galant	Birth-4-8 mos	Stroke infant's side and hips swing to that side
Moro	Birth-304 mos	Arms extend, fingers fan. If asymmetrical, suspect brrachial plexus injury. If this persists beyond 6 mos, suspect brain damage
Palmar grasp	Birth-4 mos (up to 12 mos during sleep)	Put finger in from ulnar side
Rooting	Birth-4 mos (7 mos during sleep)	Stroke corner of mouth and cheek, head turns in that direction
Sucking	B-4 mos (7 mos during sleep),	Reflexive sucking to stimuli

ASSESSMENT OF SEXUAL DEVELOPMENT (TANNER STAGES)

Male Sexual Development: The first reliable sign of sexual maturity in males is a noticeable increase in the size of the testes. This begins from ages 9 1/2 to 13 1/2. Then pubic hair appears followed by growth of the penis. Maturation from preadolescent to adult occurs over an average of 3 years.

Tanner describes 5 stages. Two separate ratings are recorded; one for pubic hair and one for genitalia.

Stage	Pubic Hair	Genitalia	
		Penis	Testes/Scrotum
I	Preadolescent. No public hair except for fine hair like that on abdomen.	Preadolescent. Same size as in childhood.	Preadolescent. Same size as in childhood.
II	Sparse, long, straight or slightly curled hair mostly at base of penis.	Slight or no enlargement.	Larger testes and scrotum, may be reddened with altered texture.
III	Darker, coarser, public hair which is curly and spread over public symphysis.	Larger, especially in length.	Further enlarged.
IV	Coarse and curly. More area covered than in Stage 3. Hair not yet on thighs.	More enlarged in length and breadth with glans development.	Further enlarged with darkened skin on scrotum.
V	Quality and quantity of adult hair which spreads to medial thigh surfaces but not over the abdomen.	Adult in size and shape.	Adult in size and shape.

Female Sexual Development: The Tanner stages are based upon external examination. Specifically, one assesses the growth of pubic hair and the development of breast tissue. Sequence of stage 2 to 5 takes an average of 3 years. Axillary hair develops approximately 2 years after pubic hair. Menarche usually occurs during breast stage 3 or 4.

Stage	Breasts	Pubic Hair
I	Preadolescent. Nipple elevation only. No elevation of underlying breast tissue.	Preadolescent. No public hair except for fine body hair similar to that on abdomen.
II	Breast buds develop. Elevation of both breast and nipple. Aureole diameter enlarges.	Sparse, long, straight or slightly curled public hair especially along labia.
III	Further enlargement and elevation of breast and aureole but no separation of their contours.	Darker, coarser, curlier hair spread sparsely over public symphysis.
IV	Aureole and nipple project forming secondary mound above breast level.	Coarse, curly pubic hair as in adults. Area covered greater than that in Stage 3 but not as great as adult. No hair yet on thighs.
V	Mature. Projection of nipple only. Aureole recedes to general contour of breast.	Adult hair in quantity and quality. Spread to medial thigh surfaces but not up over abdomen.

NEONATAL VARIANCES IN ASSESSMENT

General

Note overall impression (alert, awake, sleepy, responsive.

Note cry-intensity and pitch. High pitched cry associated with increased intacranial pressure.

Skin

Color (assess before disturbing)

> Plethoric—ruddy red color associated with a high Hematocrit.
>
> Acrocyanosis—cyanosis of the hands and feet that is normal in first few days.
>
> Jaundice—yellow color, assess in natural light, normal after first 24 hours.
>
> Bruising—common with difficult deliveries. Facial bruising common in face presentations and infants with nuchal cords.
>
> Petechiae—normal on face and upper trunk in rapid deliveries
>
> Cyanosis—assess for cause
>
> Pustular melanosis—small pustules at birth that reveal freckles when burst. Common finding in black infants and persists about 3-4 months.
>
> Erythema Toxicum—normal newborn rash. Most common in fair skinned infants. Usually appears after first 24 hours and lasts up to 2 weeks. Evanescent rash characterized by small yellow pustules on an erythematous base.
>
> Milia—small white dots usually present on nose and/or chin. Caused by blocked sweat glands. Resolve by 2-3 months.
>
> Nevus Flammeus—"Stork Bites"—also called salmon patches. Most commonly on the nape of the neck and eyelids. Turn bright red when infant cries, fade usually over the first year.
>
> Mongolian spots—normal hyperpigmented areas most commonly seen in dark skinned infants. Usually on sacral area, but can be anywhere. May be purple, blue, greenish, or brown in color.

Hair

Note whorls, abnormal coloring or distribution.

Nails

May be meconium stained. The longer the nails, the more mature the infant.

Head

Note anterior and posterior fontanelles. May appear larger than normal due to open sagittal or frontal sutures and is not of concern if FOC is normal. Sutures may be overriding due to molding to fit in birth canal. Sutures should be flat by 6 months.

> Caput Succedaneum—diffuse swelling usually over occiput that crosses suture lines and is usually resolved in first few days.
>
> Cephalhematoma—distinct swelling that does not cross suture lines. Caused by bleeding into the periosteum. Calcifies then absorbs. Persists about 3-4 months. Measure FOC and plot to determine micro or hydrocephaly. Note electrodes marks and observe them daily for infection.
>
> Craniotabes—a ping-pong ball effect of the bone usually due to thin cranial bones. Normal especially near the sutures.

Neck

Usually short. Note webbing (common in Turner's syndrome) and nuchal folds (a normal variation in large infants or associated with other findings in Down syndrome).

Ears

Note position. Low set ears associated with renal abnormalities and hearing loss. Rolled or flat helix usually due to intrauterine position. Assess for gross hearing. Newborns will blink to loud noises (Acoustical Blink Reflex).

Note preauricular pits and tags. Pits usually not significant but large tags can be associated with hearing problems.

Eyes

Note position and alignment. Note red reflex bilaterally. Cloudy red reflex associated with congenital cataracts. White reflexes associated with retinoblastoma. Red reflexes in dark skinned infants are not bright red but are a more pinkish-gray due to pigment. Lids may be puffy due to chemical conjunctivitis caused by prophylactic drops given at birth.

Short palpebral fissures may be associated with fetal alcohol syndrome.

Face

May be asymmetrical due to intrauterine position. Assess for symmetry of movement, especially if forceps were used during delivery.

Note abnormal faces.

Nose

May be asymmetrical due to position. Assess for patency. Infants obligate nose breathers until 3 months.

Mouth

Assess palate, suck,and gag. Note any natal teeth. Large tongue may be associated with hypothyroidism and Down syndrome. Note any ankyloglossia (tongue-tie). May interfere with successful breast feeding if tongue is too tightly anchored to floor of mouth.

Thorax and Lungs

Breast engorgement with or without milky discharge is normal and associated with maternal hormones. Resolves without intervention at around 2-3 weeks.

Supranumary nipples common. These will not further develop.

A newborn's xiphoid process curves upward and is normally very prominent. Breath sounds should be equal bilaterally and usually sound louder due to a thin chest wall. Note tachypnea (RR80), grunting, flaring, and retractions.

Cardiovascular
Assess as with older child. Grade II-III/VI murmurs are common at the upper LSB and if sound continuous are usually a patent ductus. Systolic murmurs at the upper left sternal border are usually transient and benign. Murmurs at the mid or lower left sternal border bear watching. Compare brachial and femoral pulses. If femoral pulses are diminished or absent, check and compare four extremity blood pressures.

Abdomen
The cord should have 3 vessels, 2 arteries and 1 vein. The cord should be treated with alcohol and should dry and fall off within the first 3 weeks. Umbilical hernias are present in 90% of newborns and are normal. Note size of defect in abdominal wall. Rectus muscle may not be fused at birth and infant has diastasis recti. This is a normal finding and will close by itself over the first year. Liver normally palpated at the costal margin but it is normal to be palpated up to half way to the umbilicus. Spleen is not normally palpated.

Anus
Check patency.

GU
Male—foreskin normally tight and meatus not visualized. Testes may be retractile or in the canals.
Female—Hypertrophied hymen or hymenal tag due to maternal hormones is common. Will recede as hormone influence fades. Also may have clear vaginal discharge that turns white, then bloody like a period before it goes away. Once resolved, it should not return. Labia minora prominent in preterm females.

Lymphatic
Nodes usually not palpable.

Musculoskeletal
Feel for crepitus over clavicles. Fractures common in large infants. With asymmetrical Moro suspect brachial plexus injury.

Feel all long bones for crepitus. Note tone. "Floppy" babies with markedly decreased tone need to be assessed further for hypoglycemia, perinatal drug exposure, sepsis, and/or chromosomal abnormalities.

Extra digits on hands originating at second knuckle of the fifth digit are very common in black infants.

Nervous System
Check normal infant reflexes. Jittery infants need to be assessed for hypoglycemia and perinatal drug exposure.

NORMAL VITAL SIGNS
Normal temperatures in children:

Age	Temperature	
	F	(C)
3 months	99.4	(37.5)
6 months	99.5	(37.5)
1 year	99.7	(37.7)
3 years	99.0	(37.2)
5 years	98.6	(37.0)
7 years	98.3	(36.8)
9 years	98.1	(36.7)
11 years	98.0	(36.7)
13 years	97.8	(36.6)

$$F = (C \times 9/5) + 32$$
$$C = (F - 32) \times 5/9$$

(adapted from Whaley and Wong, Essentials of Pediatric Nursing, 4th ed., St. Louis: Mosby Year Book, 1993)

Normal heart rates in children:

Age	Awake at rest	Asleep	Exercise/Fever
Newborn	100-180 bmp	80-160	up to 220
1 week to 3 mo	100-220 bmp	80-200	up to 220
3 mo to 2 years	80-150 bmp	70-120	up to 200
2 yr to 10 yr	70-110 bmp	60-90	up to 200
10 yr to adult	55-90 bmp	50-90	up to 200

(adapted from Whaley and Wong, Essentials of Pediatric Nursing, 4th ed., St. Louis: Mosby Year Book, 1993)

Grading of pulses:

Grade	Description
0	Not palpable
+1	Difficult to palpate; thready; weak; can be easily obliterated with pressure
+2	Difficult to palpate; may be obliterated with pressure
+3	Easy to palpate; not easily obliterated
+4	Strong; bounding; not obliterated with pressure

Normal respiratory rates for children:

Age	Rate (breaths per minute)
Newborn	35
1 to 11 mo	30
2 years	25
4 years	23
6 years	21
8 years	20
10 to 12 years	19
14 years	18
16 years	17
18 years	16-18

(adapted from Whaley and Wong, Essentials of Pediatric Nursing, 4th ed., St. Louis: Mosby Year Book, 1993)

Assessment of Normal Breath Sounds:

Classification	Description
Vesicular Breath Sounds	Heard over entire lung surface, except upper intrascapular area and area below manubrium.
Bronchovesicular Breath Sounds	Heard over manubrium and in upper intrascapular areas where trachea and bronchi bifurcate. Inspirations are louder and higher in pitch than in vesicular breathing.
Bronchial Breath Sounds	Heard only near suprasternal notch over trachea. The inspiratory phase is shorter while expiratory phase is long.

Normal Blood Pressure Rates in Children (based upon 50th percentile):

	Females		Males	
Age	Systolic	Diastolic	Systolic	Diastolic
1 day	65	55	73	55
3 days	72	55	74	55
7 days	78	54	76	54
1 mo	84	52	86	52
2 mo	87	51	91	50
3 mo	90	51	91	50
4 mo	90	52	91	50
5 mo	91	52	91	52
6 mo	91	53	90	53
7 mo	91	53	90	54
8 mo	91	53	90	55
9 mo	91	54	90	55
10 mo	91	54	90	56
11 mo	91	54	90	56
1 yr	91	54	90	56
2 yr	90	56	91	56
3 yr	91	56	92	55
4 yr	92	56	93	56
5 yr	94	56	95	56
6 yr	96	57	96	57
7 yr	97	58	97	58
8 yr	99	59	99	60
9 yr	100	61	101	61
10 yr	102	62	102	62
11 yr	105	64	105	63
12 yr	107	66	107	64
13 yr	109	64	109	63
14 yr	110	67	112	64

	Females		Males	
Age	Systolic	Diastolic	Systolic	Diastolic
15 yr	111	67	114	65
16 yr	112	67	117	67
17 yr	112	66	119	69
18 yr	112	66	121	70

(adapted from Whaley and Wong, Essentials of Pediatric
Nursing, 4th ed., St. Louis: Mosby Year Book, 1993.)

GROWTH MEASUREMENTS

One of the most important areas for assessing children is the measurement of physical growth. The pediatric nurse should measure weight, height/length, head circumference, skinfold thickness, and arm circumference. Measurements are plotted on growth charts to determine percentiles in order to compare an individual child's measurements to that of the general population.

The National Center for Health Statistics (NCHS) have developed growth charts according to age. There is one growth chart to be used for children birth to 36 months old. In this age group, the weight by age, recumbent length by age, weight for length, and head circumference by age are plotted. There is another growth chart to be used for children 2 to 18 years old. In this age group, weight by age and stature by age are plotted (see attached charts).

The National Center for Health Statistics use the 5th and 95th percentile as the parameters for determining if children fall outside of the normal limits for growth. Those below the 5th percentile are considered underweight and/or small in stature and those above the 95th percentile are considered overweight and/or large in stature. Children whose measurements fall below or above the 95th percentile should be followed more closely especially when genetic factors are not involved.

Recumbent length should be measured anytime the birth to 36 month growth chart is being used. The nurse should fully extend the infant and/or child's body. The child should be placed upon a papered surface and the nurse should mark the measurements at the top of the head and the heel of the foot. The child is then removed from the surface and measurement with a tape measure can occur.

Height is measured when using the 2 to 18 year growth chart. Height refers to the measurement taken when a child is standing upright. The child's shoes should be removed when measuring height. The head should be in midline and the child should be facing straight forward. There should be no flexion of the knees, slumping of the shoulders, or raising of the heels during the measurement. Most accurate measurements are done by using a wall mounted stadiometer.

The nurse should use a balanced scale to measure a child's weight. Children should be weighed nude when using the birth to 36 month growth chart. If a child is wearing something heavy such as a cast or an IV board that should be documented with the child's weight. When using an infant scale the nurse must remember safety issues when placing the child on this type of scale.

Head circumference is another key growth measurement in children. Generally, head circumference is measured from birth to 36 months. The measurement should be taken at the greatest circumference which is slightly above the eyebrows and ear pinna and around the occipital prominence at the back of the skull. A paper tape measure should be used to give the most accurate data.

Chest circumference is measured primarily for comparison with head circumference. Chest circumference is measured at the nipple line midway between inspiration and expiration.

The measurement of skinfold thickness is one way to assess body fat. Calipers are used to measure the skinfold thickness in one or more of the following sites: triceps, subscapula, abdomen, upper thigh, and suprailiac. An average of at least two measurements taken from each site is used.

The measurement of arm circumference is an indirect assessment used to evaluate nutrition. The arm circumference is measured with a paper tape measure. The tape is placed vertically along the posterior upper arm until the same measurement appears at the acromial process and olecranon process.

NORMAL GROWTH PARAMETERS RELATED TO WEIGHT, HEIGHT, AND HEAD CIRCUMFERENCE:

Age	Weight	Height	Head Circumference
1-6 mos	Gains 5-8 oz per week	Grows 1 in per month	
7-12 mos	Gains 4-5 oz per week	Grows 1/2 in per month	
12-18 mos	Gains 2-6 lb in next 6 mo Avg. wt is 20-24 lb. Triples birth weight by 12 mos	Grows to 33 inches by 18 months	Head circumference equals chest circum. at 12 months
18mo-3 yr	Avg wt is 28-30 lb. Quadruples birth wt by 2 yrs	Growth to 33-37 in. Approx 50% of adult height by 2 years	
3-6 yrs	Avg wt is 44 lbs	Growth to 44 inches. Doubles birth length by 4 yrs old. Ht and wt are even at 5 yrs	
7-11 yrs	Gains 5-7 lb per year	Growth appears in spurts. Increases 3 inches per year to 52 inches at 7-10 years old	

NUTRITIONAL ASSESSMENT

Nutritional status reflects the general health of a child and has a direct influence on a child's growth, development, cognition, and learning. There are many factors which affect nutrition. The nutritional assessment should consist of examining factors which affect nutrition, a dietary history, physical exam, and biochemical analysis.

Birth history should be obtained by the nurse. A history of prematurity or small gestational age is significant as it may have implications for current nutritional needs and/or problems. Past medical history especially as related to gastrointestinal disturbances should be assessed as many of these common conditions might affect nutrient intake, growth, retention, and absorption. Emotional problems can also affect nutrient intake.

It is very important to determine what medications the child is taking. Many medications affect absorption, metabolism, and excretion of nutrients. For example, antibiotics may cause decreased Vitamin K synthesis and reduce lactose, folate, and Vitamin B_{12} levels.

Culture and religion have direct influence over nutritional patterns. Both may influence types of foods eaten and patterns of eating. Socioeconomic status also plays a role in nutrition as families of lower socioeconomic status may not have economic resources or education regarding particularly nutritious foods.

A thorough dietary history should be obtained by the nurse. Types of questions to be asked will vary with the particular age of the child. Questions related to how foods are prepared, how many meals/snacks per day, food/beverage dislikes/likes, description of the child's appetite, feeding habits, vitamin supplements, and food allergies should be asked.

The nurse should attempt to obtain a 24 hour diet recall. The child and/or parent should recall every item eaten and the approximate amount. It is important that the 24 hour recall be a typical type of day for the child. One obvious disadvantage to this assessment technique is the possibility that the recall is not particularly accurate. The nurse might ask the child and or parent to keep a food diary for several days so as to obtain a more accurate account of dietary intake.

Another aspect of the nutritional assessment is the physical exam. Inspection of the skin, hair, teeth, gums, lips, tongue, and eyes can be useful in assessing possible nutritional deficits or excesses (see attached chart for physical signs of nutritional deficits). Anthropomorphic measurements of height, weight, head circumference, skinfold thickness, and arm circumference are also an essential component of the physical exam.

Lastly, biochemical analysis is an integral component of the nutritional assessment. Blood chemistry levels of hematocrit/ hemoglobin (indications of anemias), albumin (protein malnutrition), BUN (negative nitrogen balance), creatinine (high protein intake), lead (water consumption containing lead), glucose (dehydration/acidosis), and cholesterol (dietary fat intake) should be analyzed. Normal values for these tests are located in this book.

PHYSICAL SIGNS ASSOCIATED WITH NUTRITIONAL DEFICITS

Body Part	Normal Appearance	Physical Signs	Nutritional Deficit
Hair	Shiny, not easily plucked	Dull, dry, thin, easy to fall out	Protein Calories Vit C
Face/ Skin	Uniform skin color, smooth, firm	Depigmentation, scaling of skin around nostrils	Protein Riboflavin
Eyes	Bright, clear, moist membranes	Pale conjunctiva, night blindness, corneal drying	Anemia Vit A Riboflavin Niacin
Lips	Smooth, pink, not chapped	Redness and swelling, cracking	Iron Riboflavin Niacin
Tongue	Deep red, not smooth or swollen	Glositis	Folate, Niacin, Riboflavin, Iron, Vit B_{12}
Teeth	White, no cavities	Gray, black spots, mottled, pitted, grooved	Fluoride Vit D
Gums	Red without bleeding, no swelling	Spongy, bleeding, swollen	Vit C
Glands	Face not swollen	Enlarged thyroid, enlarged parotid	Iodine Protein Carlories
Nails	Firm, pink color	Spoon shaped	Iron
Bones	Can walk and run without pain	Knock knees or bow legs	Vit D
Ears	Pliable tympanic membrane (TM)	Calcified TM	Excess Vit D

DEVELOPMENTAL ASSESSMENT

Children are at high risk for developmental delay and regression from the stress of hospitalization. In order to most appropriately interact and to encourage development, the nurse needs to be knowledgeable of normal growth and developmental milestones.

GENERAL INFORMATION

Patterns of development are sequential and predictable. Children must achieve one level before they can proceed on.

Times of speech and language development are most helpful in the determination of normalcy. Vision, hearing, and physical impairment, as well as illness and hospitalization, adversely affect the results of standardized developmental testing.

DEVELOPMENTAL CHARACTERISTICS

Infants (Birth to 1 year) Erickson's Trust vs Mistrust
Personal/Social
Consistency of care is essential to the development of trust. Signaled needs must be met promptly and consistently.
Cognitive
Learn to separate self from other objects. Development of object permanence around 9-10 months is necessary for development of self image.
Motor
Rolling over to reaching out to sitting to beginning of creeping and crawling.

Toddlers (1-3 years) Erickson's Autonomy vs Shame and Doubt
Personal/Social
A period of holding on and letting go. Beginning to tolerate some separation from the parent. Parallel play.

Temper tantrums are an expression of frustration of not being able to verbalize wants. Need rituals and a safe environment in order to develop autonomy. Use negativism in quest for autonomy.

Language/Cognitive

Major achievement is language development. Appearance denotes function. Imitates household activities. Is very egocentric.

Motor

A major skill is the development of locomotion, i.e., walking, running, climbing. A major task is toilet training. Developing pincher grasp.

Preschoolers (3-6 Years) Erickson's Initiative vs Guilt

Personal/Social

Need a security object. Are learning sex differences. Are energetic learners and feel guilt for not behaving or acting appropriately. Also may feel guilt from having thoughts that differ from the perceived norm. Beginnings of morality and the development of a conscience. Have a fear of mutilation and injury. Have poorly defined body boundaries and need a bandage to maintain body integrity.

Language/Cognitive

Talk incessantly and in complete sentences. Have global organization of thought. Changing any part of something, changes the whole thing. Give life-like qualities to inanimate objects. Cannot perceive opposite behavior so need to phrase directions positively. Are shifting from total egocentricity to beginning to be able to consider other view points. Have magical thinking and accept meaning literally.

Motor

Walking, running, climbing, jumping are well established.
Most can use scissors by age 4 years and tie shoes by 5 years.

School-Agers (6-12 years) Erickson's Industry vs Inferiority

Personal/Social

Goal is to achieve a sense of personal and interpersonal competence by acquiring technologies and social skills.

Failure to accomplish this leads to a sense of inferiority. Further development of conscience. Peer groups are influential and necessary but the parents still are the primary influence.

Language/Cognitive

Use thought processes to explore events. Can see things from other points of view. Can reason.

Adolescents (12-18 years) Erickson's Identity vs. Role Confusion

Personal/Social

Trying to develop a sense of identity. Early adolescents need peer approval. Later adolescents need autonomy from their family and develop a sense of personal identity. They need a group identity to develop a personal identity. Are on an emotional roller coaster. Body image established during adolescence is the one the individual retains throughout life.

Cognitive

They can think beyond the present. Are concerned with the possible. Use logic and scientific reasoning. Are capable of abstract thinking. Want a clear picture of life and its purposes.

DEVELOPMENTAL ASSESSMENT TOOLS

Optimum developmental screening should be done with well children. Hospitalized children may have multiple variables interfering with normal testing. There are many tools available. The most commonly used tool is the Denver II.

Although during hospitalization is not the optimum time to test children, this tool can be utilized as a quick reference for the sequencing of normal milestones and to help identify areas of stimulation that would be appropriate.

Denver II

Used to assess well children from birth to 6 years. It is designed to "compare a given child's performance on a variety of tasks to the performance of other children the same age." (Frankenburg,

1990). It is not a predictor of future development and does not test IQ.

To perform the Denver II, one must read the booklet with strict guidelines that are specific to testing and interpretation and use the kit with the materials provided. Inclusion of the example in this text is solely to aid the nurse in identification of areas of development to encourage stimulation of in order to help minimize developmental delay and regression.

R-PDQ Revised Prescreening Developmental Questionnaire
Assesses children birth to 6 years. Is a parent answered prescreening based on questions from the DDST. Four different forms are available based on age. This gives the parent's perspective of the child's developmental abilities.

(Both of the above tests with forms and complete instructions
are available from Denver Developmental Materials, Inc.,
P.O. Box 6919, Denver, CO 80206-9019).

PLAY ASSESSMENT

Play is described as the 'work' of children. It is crucial to maintain the activities of play with hospitalized children.

Suggested Play Activities For Hospitalized Children

Infants — colorful mobiles, music boxes, mirrors, infant swing, "patty cake"

Toddlers — singalong tapes, pull toys, riding toys

Preschool — puppet making, favorite character videos, drawing/coloring, cutting out pictures

SchoolAge — card playing, "hangman", drawing, favorite movie videos, video games, encourage peer interaction

Adolescent — board games, audio tapes, radio, video movies, mental challenge games, craft activities

Therapeutic Play is used when the child is unable to verbalize their feelings. It is used to better understand the child's thoughts about hospitalization, procedures, fears, and concerns. Both verbal and nonverbal messages from the child are important. Drawing, painting, using anatomically-correct dolls, and direct play with medical equipment are often used.

Therapeutic Play Guidelines

a. Allow as much choice as possible for child in selecting articles to play with.

b. Allow child to play with actual medical materials that he/she will be confronted with (i.e., stethoscope, NG tube, tympanic thermometer).

c. Utilize therapeutic communication techniques.

d. Ask child to describe his/her drawings.

e. Therapeutic play should always be supervised.

PAIN ASSESSMENT

Factors That Affect Children's Response to Pain

Culture
Developmental level
Parental attitudes
Expectation
Education/Teaching
Anesthesia/Type of procedure
Previous experience with pain
Parent's presence or absence
Nurse's/Doctor's attitudes and beliefs about pain
Fear

Physical signs & symptoms (possible)

Facial expression of discomfort/Grimacing
Immobility
Elevated pulse/Respirations
Irritability/Restlessness
Decreased appetite

Developmental Responses

Infants
Irritability, crying, withdrawal, pushing away, restless sleeping
Toddlers
Very quiet, regressive behavior, uncooperative, crying, point to where it hurts, say ooww, fear responses. (May leave room to go to safe area of the playroom even though he hurts because the fear of what will happen to him in his room overshadows his pain.)
Preschoolers
Become quiet, may feel its punishment for bad behavior or thoughts. Good at procrastination before painful procedures. (persistent "Wait a minute" or "I have to go to the bathroom")

May be able to tell where it hurts and use tools to describe the severity.

Schoolagers

May deny pain to be brave or to avoid further hurt. Withdraw, watch or stare at the TV.

Adolescents

Fear loss of control. Are affected by mood changes and expectations of behavior. May refuse or over request medication. Show increased muscle tension.

Assessment Guidelines

Assess frequently and uniformly using age appropriate tools and nursing observations. Tools help to more accurately assess and record pain assessment and need to be used and recorded at least once a shift. This provides a record to see if pain is increasing or decreasing and if relief methods are effective.

Pain Assessment Tools

Wong/Baker Faces Scale

Used with ages 3-10 years.

Numeric scale (0-10)—0 is no hurt, 10 is worst hurt ever had. Child picks a number between 0 and 10 to describe the severity of hurt. Has to know numbers and works best with 5 year olds and older.

Poker Chip Tool—Uses 5 poker chips to measure pieces of hurt. Works with 4 year olds and older.

Color tool—uses outline of body and child chooses a color to indicate the degree of hurt and colors where it hurts.

Need to consult hospital policy regarding tools used in that facility and read original information and guidelines to use tool chosen.

SIGNS AND SYMPTOMS OF DRUG EXPOSURE/USE

Neonatal Exposure

Symmetrical growth retardation, decreased weight and/FOC

Poor response to auditory and visual stimuli, may be sleepy and/or easily overstimulated and become irritable.

Poor feeding vs hyperphagia

Vomiting/diarrhea

Sweating

Excessive crying

Jittery/tremors

Hyperreflexia/increased muscle tone vs decreased muscle tone

Frantic hand sucking

Pallor

Drug Use

Physical Signs & Symptoms (And Possible Drugs Associated With)
Headache (Inhalants)
Hyperreflexia (Cocaine, Hallucinogens)
Hyporeflexia (Narcotics, Heroin)
Slurred speech, Ataxia (Alcohol)
Bulky Muscles (Steroids)
Jaundice (Alcohol)
Tachycardia, Elevated BP (Alcohol, Cocaine, Hallucinogens)
Bradycardia, Decreased BP (Heroin, Narcotics)

Chest Pain (Cocaine)
Increased Respirations (Cocaine)
Decreased Respirations (Alcohol, Heroin, Narcotics)
Rhinorrhea (Alcohol)
Erythematous Nasal Septum (Cocaine, Inhalants)
Epistaxis (Cocaine)
Red/Bloodshot Eyes/Conjunctivitis (Alcohol, Marijuana, Inhalants)
Dilated Pupils (Cocaine)
Constricted Pupils (Heroin, Narcotics)
Needle Marks (Heroin, Narcotics)

Social Signs & Symptoms
Multiple Accidents
Multiple STD's
Aggressive Behavior
Antisocial Behavior

Psychological Signs & Symptoms
Depression
Anxiety
Sleep Changes
Hallucinations
Euphoria
Mood Changes (Excessive)
Memory Loss/Blackouts

CHILD ABUSE ASSESSMENT

FAILURE TO THRIVE

Characterized by lack of normal growth and development.
Usually affects those 18 months and younger.
Weight is below the 5th percentile.
Are irritable, resist cuddling, and are unresponsive to nurturing.
Appear thin, frail, undernourished, with big, vacant eyes.

May have gaze aversion.

Have drawn, pinched, anxious or expressionless face. Usually will not smile.

Are obsessed with thumb or pacifier.

Will usually gain weight in hospital on same formula was on at home.

PHYSICAL

Characterized by certain types of behaviors and injuries.

Behaviors

Parent	Child
Delay in seeking treatment	Withdrawn
Variation in history	Doesn't cry or respond to
Injury doesn't fit history	painful procedures
Unable to comfort child	May accuse adult
Absence of accused parent	May try to console parent
Decreased visits	
Lack of follow through	
Blames sibling or patient	

Injuries Suspicious of Abuse

Bruises over soft tissue areas
Multiple planes of bruises
Multiple ages of bruises

Dating of bruises (related to Hgb breakdown)

0-2 days	swollen and tender
0-5 days	red-blue
5-7 days	greenish yellow
7-10 days	yellow to brown
10-14 days	brown
2-4 weeks	clear

Bilateral black eyes including upper lids
Slap, grab marks

Human bite marks with greater than 3 cm between canines (adult teeth)

Linear bruises from belt

Bruises shaped like the object used to inflict them

Tie marks on extremities

Gag marks

Cigarette burns

Dry contact burns that are second degree

Forced emersion burns (dunking or donut burns) Usually spare the buttocks and feet because they were held against the cool bottom of the tub, have no splash marks, and a clear line of demarcation between burned and unburned areas of skin.

Stocking or glove burns with no splash marks, are clearly demarcated, and go above the ankle or the wrist.

Subdural hematomas with retinal hemorrhages from a shaking injury.

Boggy scalp due to subgaleal hematoma caused by lifting the scalp off the skull.

Traumatic alopecia—hair loss with tender scalp and broken hairs around patch of missing hair.

Spiral fractures of the humerus or femur from a twisting injury.

Fractured ribs in an infant.

Bucket Handle fractures of femur or humerus.

Signs of Sexual Abuse

Usually few physical signs but may see the following:
    Abdominal and/or genital bruising
    Lacerations of vagina or rectum
    Sexually transmitted diseases in prepubertal child
    Irritation or pain
    Pregnancy
Behavioral Signs
    Advanced knowledge of explicit sexual behavior
    Sexual acting out
    Withdrawal

Fear of adult males/females

Depression

Encopresis (Incontinence of stool)

Enuresis (Incontinence of urine)

Run away behaviors

Child's story—often is the only evidence. Nurse must believe the child. They need support and most importantly, need to know that it was not in any way their fault. The guilt is tremendous and they need praise for having the courage to tell.

Munchausen's Syndrome by Proxy

Child's signs and symptoms cannot be explained by known disease etiologies

Tests, x-rays, and studies are negative

Child has repeated hospitalizations for the same problem

Mom's history is unsupported by other caretakers

Child improves when mom is not present

Possible positive family history, especially siblings for same problems

Child usually 6 years old or younger

Father absent or uninvolved

Mom overinvolved and has some type of experience in health care

BURNS ASSESSMENT

I.   Epidemiology: Second most common cause of death from trauma in childhood. Children under 4 years of age are at greatest risk. Burns frequently occur between the hours of 6pm and midnight. Incidence is often related to the quality and quantity of adult supervision.

II.   Etiology: Burns can be caused by thermal, chemical, electrical, or radioactive injuries.

III. Extent of injury: The amount of tissue destroyed determines the physiologic responses, therapy, and prognosis for the injured child. The severity of the injury is based upon the percentage of body surface burned, depth of the burn, and the location of the burn.

    A. Burn Assessment: Calculate the child's body surface area.

        1. Burn depth (can change over first several days)

            a. First degree: only epidermis involved, characterized by pain and erythema

            b. Second degree: epidermis and dermis involved with dermal appendages spared, may be blistered and painful if superficial or white and painless if deep

            c. Third degree: full-thickness burns involving epidermis and all of dermis (including appendages), painless, require grafting

        2. Burn Assessment Chart: Used to map out areas of second and third degree burns and to calculate the total BSA burned.

            a. The rule of nines: See figure. Because of body proportions, especially the head and lower extremities, the 'rule of nines' are not applicable to children younger than 10 years old. Must modify % BSA burned using Lund-Browder chart.

            b. Lund-Browder chart: See figure page 56

Relative percentage of areas affected by growth

Back	At birth	Age 1	Age 5	Age 10
A Half of head	9 1/2%	8 1/2%	6 1/2%	5 1/2%
B. Half of thigh	2 3/4%	3 1/4%	4%	4 1/4%
C. Half lower leg	2 1/2%	2 1/2%	2 3/4%	3o%

	Age 15
A. Half of head	4 1/2%
B. Half of thigh	4 1/2%
C. Half of lower leg	3 1/4%

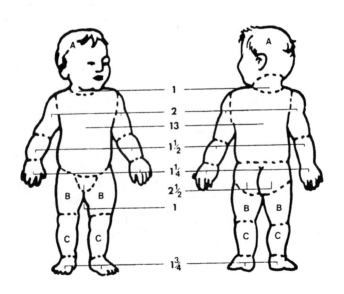

CLINICAL VALUES AND STANDARDS

CLINICAL VALUES AND STANDARDS
TABLE OF CONTENTS

CALCULATING CALORIC REQUIREMENTS IN CHILDREN

Age	Daily Requirements
High-risk neonate	120-150 calories/kg/day
Normal neonate	100-120 calories/kg/day
1-2 years	90-100 calories/kg/day
2-6 years	80-90 calories/kg/day
7-9 years	70-80 calories/kg/day
10-12 years	50-60 calories/kg/day

(Children with disease, surgery, fever, or pain may require additional calories above the maintenance value. Comatose or immobile children may require less.)

(adapted from Mary Fran Hazinski, *Nursing Care of the Critically Ill Child*, 2 ed., 1992. St. Louis: Mosby Year Book.)

CALCULATION OF MAINTENANCE FLUIDS IN CHILDREN

Child's Weight	Kilogram body-weight formula
Newborns 0-72 hrs old)	60-100 ml/kg
0-19 kg	100 ml/kg
11-20 kg	1000 ml for the first 10 kg plus 50 ml/kg for each kg over 10 kg
21-30 kg	1500 ml for the first 20 kg plus 25 ml/kg for each kg over 20 kg

Urine output should average 0.5 to 1.0 ml/kg/hour when child's fluid intake is adequate.

(adapted from Mary Fran Hazinski, *Nursing Care of the Critically Ill Child*, 2 ed., 1992. St. Louis: Mosby Year Book.)

NORMAL LAB VALUES AND INTERPRETATION

ALT (SGPT)

Infant	6u/L
Child/Adult	1-45u/L

Increased in severe hepatitis, infectious mononucleosis, CHF, eclampsia. Not as specific for liver function as AST.

AST (SGOT)

Newborn/Infant	20-65u/L
Child/Adult	0-35u/L

Increased in liver necrosis, Reyes syndrome. Not likely to be decreased.

BICARBONATE (HCO$_3$)

Infant	20-24mEq/L
2 years	22-26mEq/L

Functions as a buffer to keep normal pH. Increased in metabolic alkalosis. Decreased in metabolic acidosis.

BILIRUBIN (TOTAL)   DIRECT (BC)

Term Infants   < 0.2mg/dl

0-1day	< 6mg/dl
1-2days	< 8mg/dl
3-7days	< 12mg/dl
> 1 month	0.2-1mg/dl
Adult	0.1-1mg/dl

INDIRECT (BU)
Total-direct = indirect
(Total-BC = BU)

BU (bilirubin unconjugated) is increased in any condition that causes hemolysis of red blood cells.

BC(bili conjugated) is increased in conditions that cause obstruction in normal bile flow.

BLOOD UREA NITROGEN (BUN)

5-25mg/dl

Used primarily to assess renal function but is affected by protein breakdown, hydration, and liver failure. Increased in severe dehydration and impaired renal perfusion. Decreased in overhydration.

CALCIUM-TOTAL SERUM (CA)

< 1 week	7-12mg/dl
child	8-10.5mg/dl

Increased in dehydration, Vitamin D intoxication, and metastatic bone disease. Decreased in chronic renal disease, severe malnutrition, and with low albumin levels.

CHLORIDE (Cl)

94-106mEq/L.

Increases as sodium increases. Decreases commonly due to loss from vomiting, diarrhea, and diuretics.

CHOLESTEROL

Infant	53-135mg/dl
Child	70-175mg/dl
Adolescent	120-210mg/dl
Adult	140-250mg/dl

35mg/dl HDL (High density lipid) "good cholesterol"
nmg/dl LDL (Low density lipid) "bad cholesterol"

Increased in those with diet high in cholesterol and saturated fats. Some also have a genetic predisposition. Decreased in hyperthyroidism, severe liver damage, and malnutrition.

COMPLETE BLOOD COUNT (CBC)

Red blood cells (RBC)

Newborn	5.5-6 million/mm3
Child	4.6-4.8 million/mm3
Adult male	4.6-5.9 million/mm3
female	4.2-5.4 million/mm3

Increased number in high altitudes, increased physical strain, chronic lung disease, and cyanotic heart disease. Decreased due to abnormal loss or destruction and bone marrow suppression.

DESCRIPTORS

hypochromic—less color
normochromic—normal color
microcytic—small size
normocytic—normal size
macrocytic—large size

Hemoglobin (Hgb, Hb)

Newborn	17-19gm
Child	14-17gm
Adult male	13-18gm
female	12-16gm

If increased, look at in relation to the number and size of RBC's. Decreased in all conditions that cause a decrease in RBC's. (Abnormal hemoglobin, increased fragility leading to increased destruction.

Hematocrit (Hct)

Newborn	up to 65%	
Child (mean)		
2 weeks	53%	
1 month	44%	
2 months	35%	
6 months-2 years		36%
2-6 years	37%	
6-12 years		40%
12-18 years male		43%
female		41%
Adult male		45-52%
female		37-48%

Is the percent of RBC's in plasma. Is roughly three times the Hgb. Capillary values may be 5-10% higher than vena puncture. Increased in normally hydrated child indicates a true increase in RBC's. Can be increased in dehydration and decreased in over hydration.

Mean Corpuscular Volume (MCV)

Newborn   95-121μm3
6-24 months   70-86μm3
gradually increases to 78-98μm3
Describes the average size of an individual RBC.

Hct $\div$ RBC = MCV

If less than 86μm3 are microcytic and possibly indicates iron deficiency anemia, lead poisoning, or thalassemia. Greater than 98μm3 are macrocytic and possible pernicious anemia or folic acid deficiency.

Mean Corpuscular Hemoglobin (MCH)

27-32pg
Amount of Hgb in a single cell.

$Hgb \div RBC = MCH$

Mean Corpuscular Hemoglobin Concentration (MCHC)

32-36%

Proportion of each cell occupied by Hgb.

RBC Distribution Width (RDW)

11.5-14.5%

Variation of cell width. May help assess types of anemias. Iron deficiency anemia increases the RDW, thalassemia does not.

Platlets (Plt)

Newborn	100,000-290,000/mm3
Child	150,000-350,000/mm3
Adult	150,000-350,000/mm3

Have an 8-10 day life span. Aid in coagulation by adhering and clumping. Increased (thrombocytosis) in malignancy and polycythemia. Decreased (thrombocytopenia) in ITP, after viral illness, in AIDS, bone marrow suppression, and with patients with enlarged spleens destroying them too fast.

White Blood Cells (WBC)

Newborn	10,000-35,000
Child	8,000-14,500
Adult	4,300-10,000

Total white blood cell count. Increased in bacterial infection, and leukemias, especially acute lymphocytic leukemia. Decreased in bone marrow suppression, overwhelming sepsis, and with certain chemotherapy.

Differential (Diff)

	Segs	Bands	Lymph	Mono	Baso	Eos
NB	50-60%	3-5%	30-40%	3-7%	0-1%	0-3%
6m	32%		61%			
1-2y	31-33%		59-61%			
4y	42%		50%			
6y	51%	42%				
8-21y	53-59%		34-39%	4-5%		

Percent must add up to 100%. Left shift is usually seen in bacterial infections. The left side of the differential (Segs and bands) increases. Segs and bands are neutrophils. Left shift may also be calculated as an immature to total (IT) neutrophil ratio of .20 or greater.

IT = Bands (Immature) ÷ Bands and Segs (Total) = .20

ANC (Absolute Neutrophil Count) = %segs + %bands × # of WBC's

    Ex.: WBC count =10,000   Segs=51% Bands=2%

    51% + 2% = 53%   10,000 X 53% = ANC of 5,300

Segs—Segmented neutrophils, mature form

Bands—immature form

Are increased in bacterial infections, inflammatory processes, and tissue necrosis. Are decreased (neutropenia) in viral diseases, hepatitis, influenza, measles, mumps, and rubella, and overwhelming infections.

Lymph—lymphocytes

Principal component of the immune system.

T lymphocyte is about 60-80%
B lymphocyte is about 5-15%
Non T, Non B is about 10-20%
Are increased in viral infections, mumps, hepatitis, retrovirus, mono, tumors, and TB. Markedly increased in lymphocytic leukemias. Decreased in AIDS, severe malnutrition, and in any condition that increases the neutrophils.

Mono—monocytes
Increase usually due to chronic conditions such as TB, malaria, and Rocky Mountain Spotted Fever.

Baso—Basophils
Increased in malignancy.

Eos—eosinophils
Increased in allergic reactions, asthma, drug reactions, and parasitic infections. Decreased in corticosteroid use.

CREATININE (SERUM)

Newborn	0.3-1mg/dl
Infant	0.2-0.4mg/dl
Child	0.3-0.7mg/dl
Adolescent	0.5-1mg/dl

Used only to evaluate renal function. Does not increase until at least half the nephrons are nonfunctioning.

FERRITIN

20-400ng/L

Directly related to the amount of iron in storage. Increased in chronic illness, malignancy, and chronic transfusions. Decreased in malnutrition.

GLUCOSE

Term   40-110mg/dl
1 week-16 years   60-105mg/dl
Adult   70-110mg/dl

Most common reason for persistent increase is diabetes mellitus.
Mild diabetic acidosis   300-450mg/dl
Moderate diabetic acidosis   450-600mg/dl
Severe diabetic acidosis   600mg/dl and up
Decreased with too little food intake and increased exercise.
Spills into the urine when blood glucose in 160-190mg/dl.

IRON (SERUM)

Newborn	100-250mcg/dl
Infant	40-100mcg/dl
Child	50-120mcg/dl
Adolescent	
Male	50-160mcg/dl
Female	40-150mcg/dl
Adult	50-150mcg/dl (male slightly increased)

Evening levels are lower so draw in morning. Should have no iron
supplements for 24 hours before test. Decreased in iron deficiency
anemia.

LEAD (Pb)

Class
I	9mcg/dl or less	Low risk, retest at 2 years of age.
IIA	10-14mcg/dl	Borderline, retest every 3-4 mos until have 3 results less than 15mcg/dl, then test annually.
IIB	15-19mcg/dl	Retest every 3-4 months.

III	20-44mcg/dl	Need medical evaluation. Test for iron deficiency anemia. Environmental sources need to be identified and eliminated. May possibly need pharmacological treatment.
IV	45-69mcg/dl	Medical treatment, environmental assessment and remediation within 48 hours.
V	70mcg/dl or higher	Medical treatment, environmental assessment and remediation immediately. (Recommendations by the CDC)

Finger stick lead levels that are elevated need to be reconfirmed by venipuncture.

MAGNESIUM

1.5-2mEq/L

Increased in renal failure and in patients receiving IV magnesium sulfate. Decreased in chronic malnutrition, chronic aminoglycoside use and chronic hypercalcemia.

PHOSPHORUS

Newborn	4.2-9.5mg/dl
Infant	4.5-6.5mg/dl
Child	3.5-6mg/dl
Adult	2.7-4.5mg/dl

Increased in renal failure and vitamin D toxicity.
Decreased in malabsorption.
Most frequent and dangerous electrolyte disorder in hyperalimentation.

POTASSIUM (K)

3.5-5mEq/L

Elevations usually associated with inadequate renal output. Decreased usually due to loss through the GI tract from vomiting and NG tube drainage.
Small changes have a great effect on cardiac muscle. Hemolysis from squeezing finger or heel can falsely elevate results.

RETICULOCYTE COUNT (RETIC)

Newborn	3-5%
Child/Adult	0.5-2.5%

Are less mature RBC's. Measure bone marrow function.
Increases due to increased destruction and need for more RBC's from hemolysis of ABO incompatibility and sickle cell disease, or to increased loss for acute blood loss. Will increase after treatment begun for iron deficiency anemia. Decreased in abnormal bone marrow function.

SODIUM (Na)

135-145mEq/L

Changes not commonly seen because its concentration is always correlated with fluid balance. Elevated in hypertonic dehydration with loss of large amounts of water without proportional losses of sodium. Decreased in water intoxication where loss of sodium and water is replaced with only water.

TRIGLYCERIDES

Newborn	(mg/dl and rises to 55-60mg/dl
10-14 years	65-75mg/dl
15-19 years	75-80mg/dl

Increased in nephrotic syndrome, hypothyroidism and diabetes.
Decreased is rarely a problem.

URINALYSIS (UA)

Color	Light yellow to dark amber
Clarity	Should be clear
Odor	Fresh specimen should not have ammonia smell
pH	4.3-8, average 6, is affected by diet. Most bacteria (except E coli) increase the pH and create an alkaline urine.

Specific Gravity

Infants-2 years	1.001-1.018
Adult	1.001-1.040 (Usually 1.015-1.025)

If fixed at 1.010 (Sp.Gr. of plasma) the kidney has
lost the ability to concentrate urine.
The higher the number, the more concentrated the
urine.

Protein	Usually negative. Persistent proteinuria is indicative of renal dysfunction.
Sugar	Usually negative. If positive, blood glucose is at least 160 mg/dl.
Ketone	Negative. If positive, body is burning fat for energy.

Nitrites and Leukocyte esterase (LE)

Should be negative. If positive usually has UTI.

Bilirubin	Negative. If positive, is the first indication of liver disease before jaundice.
Urobilinogen	Increased in hemolytic disease.
Sediment	
Crystals	Uric acid, Calcium oxalate, and triple phosphates are normal.
Casts	Most are pathological. A few hyaline casts are normal. WBC casts (4-5) are associated with infection. RBC casts are associated with damage to the glomerular membrane.

CONVERSION TABLES FOR COMMONLY USED EQUIVALENTS

1 gram (gm)	=	1000 milligrams (mg)
1 gm	=	1 cubic centimeter (cc)
1 gm	=	15 or 16 grains (gr)
60 or 65mg	=	1 grain (gr)
1 mg	=	1000 micrograms (mcg)
1 kilogram (kg)	=	1000 gm
1 kg	=	2.2 pounds
1 milliliter (ml)	=	1 cc
1 ml	=	15 or 16 minims
1 drop (gtt)	=	1 minim
4 ml	=	1 dram (fluid dram)
5 ml	=	1 teaspoon (tsp)
15 ml	=	1 Tablespoon (Tbsp)
30 ml	=	1 ounce (fluid ounce) (oz.)
500 ml	=	1 pint (pt)
1000ml	=	1 liter (L.)
1 L.	=	1 quart (qt)
1 inch (in)	=	2.54 centimeters (cm)
1 cm	=	10 millimeters (mm)

For quick rough conversions:

Pounds to kg: subtract the first number in the pounds from the total pounds and divide by 2.
Ex. Weight= 45 pounds. 45-4=41. 41 ÷ 2 = 20.5 kg.

Inches to cm: inches × 10 ÷ 4 = cm
Ex. Length=18 inches. 18 × 10 = 180 ÷ 4 = 45 cm.

Cm. to inches: cm × 4 ÷ 10 = inches
Ex.Length=45cm. 45 × 4 ÷ 10 = 18 in.

COMMON ABBREVIATIONS IN PEDIATRIC NURSING

AIDS	Acquired Immune Deficiency Syndrome
ALT	Alanine Aminotransferase (SGPT)
ASD	Atrial Septal Defect
AST	Aspartate Aminotransferase (SGOT)
BCS	Battered Child Syndrome
BPD	Bronchopulmonary Dysplasia
BUN	Blood Urea Nitrogen
CBC	Complete Blood Count
CF	Cystic Fibrosis
CHD	Congenital Heart Disease
	Cyanotic Heart Disease
CHF	Congestive Heart Failure
CL	Central Line
COA	Coarctation of the Aorta
CP	Cerebral Palsy
CPR	Cardiopulmonary Resuscitation
CT	Computerized Tomography
CXR	Chest X-ray
DOB	Date of Birth
DTP	Diphtheria, Tetanus, Pertussis
ECD	Endocardial Cushion Defect
ECHO	Echocardiogram
EKG	Electrocardiogram
FAS	Fetal Alcohol Syndrome
FOC	Formula of Choice
	Frontal Occipital Circumference
FTT	Failure to Thrive
FUO	Fever of Unknown Origin
GER	Gastroesophageal Reflux
GI	Gastrointestinal
GTT	Glucose Tolerance Test
HIB	Haemophilus Influenzae B vaccine

IDM	Infant of a Diabetic Mother
IPV	Inactivated Polio Vaccine
IUGR	Intrauterine Growth Retardation
JDM	Juvenile Diabetes Mellitus
JRA	Juvenile Rheumatoid Arthritis
MMR	Measles, Mumps, Rubella
MR	Mental Retardation
MSBP	Munchausen's Syndrome by Proxy
NEC	Necrotizing Enterocolitis
NPO	Nothing by Mouth
OD	Right eye
OPV	Oral Polio Vaccine
OS	Left eye
OU	Each eye
PBS	Phenobarbital
PDA	Patent Ductus Arteriosus
PGG	Ph, Glucose, and Guaiac
PKU	Phenylketonuria
PPD	Purified Protein Derivative (TB skin test)
PPS	Post Pericardial Syndrome
RAD	Reactive Airway Disease
RDS	Respiratory Distress Syndrome
RMSF	Rocky Mountain Spotted Fever
ROM	Range of Motion
ROS	Rule Out sepsis
SCD	Sickle Cell Disease
SIDS	Sudden Infant Death Syndrome
SLE	Systemic Lupus Erythematosus
SO	Significant Other
STD	Sexually Transmitted Disease
TGA	Transposition of the Great Arteries
TOF	Tetralogy of Fallot
TORCH	Toxoplasmosis, Other, Rubella, Cytomegalovirus, Herpes

TPN	Total Parenteral Nutrition
UA	Urinalysis
VSD	Ventricular Septal Defect

DRUG ADMINISTRATION

DRUG ADMINISTRATION
TABLE OF CONTENTS

COMMON PEDIATRIC DRUGS

ACETAMINOPHEN

(Tylenol and others)

Indications:

Mild to moderate pain, fever.

Administer:

10-15 mg/kg/dose q4-6h, 5 doses in 24h. Max. dose: 4gm/24h
Dosing by age:
   0-3mo: 40mg/dose
   4-11mo: 80mg/dose
   12-24mo: 120mg/dose
   2-3yr: 160mg/dose
   4-5yr: 240mg/dose
   6-8yr: 320mg/dose
   9-10yr: 400mg/dose
   11-12yr: 480mg/dose
   Adult: 325-650mg/dose
   PO or suppository

Nursing Implications:

Dose standardization common. Contraindicated in known G6PD deficiency. Rectal absorption variable. Use cautiously in severe hepatic disease. Assess and document effect 30-60 minutes after administration.

ACYCLOVIR

(Zovirax)

Indications:

Treatment of Herpes simplex virus, varicella zoster.

Administer:

Herpes Simplex virus:
    Newborn: 30mg/kg/24h ÷ q8h IV
    Children yr: 250mg/m²/dose IV q8h
    Adult: 15mg/kg/24h ÷ q8h IV
Varicella Zoster:
    Children yr: 30mg/kg/24h ÷ q8h IV
    Children 1yr: 1500mg/m²/24h ÷ q8h IV
    Adult: 30mg.kg.24h ÷ q8h IV
IV Dilution:max. conc: 7-10mg/ml
    usual mg/ml over 60 min.
Compatibility: D5 (5% Dextrose), NS (Normal Saline), LR (Lactated Ringers)

Nursing Implications:

Adequate hydration and slow administration essential to prevent crystal formation in renal tubules. Dose reduction required in renal impairment. PO dosing not well established.

ALBUTEROL

(Proventil, Ventolin)

Indications:

Bronchodilator in asthma or RAD (reactive airway disease).

Administer:

Children yr: 0.3mg/kg/24h PO ÷ q8h (max. dose: 12mg/24h)
    6-11yr: 6mg/24h PO ÷ TID (max. dose: 24mg/24h)
    ≥12yr and adult: 2-4mg dose PO TID-QID (max. dose: 32mg/24h

Nursing Implications:

Administer with meals to decrease gastric irritation. Also used as an inhalant.

AMIKACIN

(Amikin)

Indications:

Treatment of serious gram negative bacillary infections and infections due to staphylococcus when penicillin and other less toxic drugs are contraindicated.

Administer:

Children and adult: 15-22.5mg/kg/24h ÷ q8-12h IV/IM
Max. dose: 1.5gm/24h
IV dilution: 5mg/ml over 30-60 min.
Compatibility: D5, NS, LR

Nursing Implications:

Therapeutic levels must be monitored. Peak: 20-30mg/L; Trough: 5-10mg/L. Dose adjusted in renal insufficiency. Patient needs to be well hydrated.

AMINOPHYLLINE

(many brands)

Indications:

Bronchodilator in reversible airway obstruction due to asthma. Also as respiratory and myocardial stimulant in apnea of infancy.

Administer:

IV loading: 6mg/kg IV over 20 min.

IV maintenance: continuous drip:

    Neonates: 0.2mg/kg/hr

    6wk-6mo: 0.5mg/kg/hr

    6mo-1yr: 0.6-0.7mg/kg/hr

    1-9yr: 1-1.2mg/kg/hr

    9-12yr and young adult smokers: 0.9mg/kg/hr

    Adult and nonsmoking young adult: 0.5mg/kg/hr

Above daily total doses can be given IV q4-6h

Neonatal apnea:

    Loading dose: 5-6mg/kg/IV or PO

    Maintenance: 1-2mg/kg/dose q6-8h IV or PO

PO:

    1-9yr: 20mg/kg/24h ÷ q4-6h

    9-16yr: 16mg/kg/24h ÷ q6h

    Adult: 12mg/kg/24h ÷ q6h

    IV dilution: Loading: 4mg/ml bolus over 20-30 min.

Continuous infusion: 0.8mg/ml

Compatibility: D5

Nursing Implications:

Must monitor for serum levels. Therapeutic levels for asthma: 10-20mg/L; for neonatal apnea: 6-13mg/L. Can cause restlessness, vomiting. arrhythmias, and seizures.

AMOXICILLIN

(Amoxil, Larotid, etc.)

Indications:

Treatment of a variety of infections including most commonly otitis media as a first line drug. Also used in sinusitis, respiratory and GU tract infections, and for SBE prophylaxis.

Administer:

Child: 20-50mg/kg/24h ÷ q8h PO
Adult: 250-500mg/dose q8h PO
Max. dose: 2gm/24h

Nursing Implications:

Most common side effects are rashes and diarrhea.

AMOXICILLIN-CLAVULANIC ACID

(Augmentin)

Indications:

Same as amoxicillin but extends its activity to include beta-lactamase producing strains of H-Influenza and B. Catarrhalis.

Administer:

Child (kg: 20-40mg/kg/24h ÷ q8h PO
Adult: 250-500mg/dose q8h PO
    Max. dose: 2gm/24h

Nursing Implications:

Incidence of diarrhea higher than with Amoxicillin. Give with meals to help decrease GI side effects.

AMPICILLIN

(Omnipen, Polycillin)

Indications:

Treatment of otitis media, sinusitis, respiratory tract infections, GU infections, meningitis, septicemia, and as endocarditis prophylaxis.

Administer:

Neonate ≥7 days and ≥2 kg: 100-200mg/kg/24h ÷ q6h IV/IM
Child:

> Mild to moderate infections: 50-100mg/kg/24h ÷ q6h
> PO/IV/IM
> Max. PO dose: 2-4gm/24h
> Severe infections: 200-400mg/kg/24h ÷ q4-6h IV/IM
> Max. IV dose: 12gm/24h

IV dilution: Direct IV up to 500mg only, max. conc. 100mg/ml
over 3-5 min.

> Intermittent infusion: 30mg/ml over 10-60min.

Compatibility: NS preferred, LR, SW (Sterile water)

Nursing Implications:

Higher doses used to treat CNS disease. Hypersensitivity rash
commonly seen at 5-10 days. Reconstituted Ampicillin Sodium
effective for one hour after reconstitution. IV administration at
greater than 100mg/min. may cause seizures.

ASPIRIN

(ASA, Anacin, Bayer, etc.)

Indications:

Mild pain, and fever. Also useful as anti-inflammatory and in
Kawasaki disease.

Administer:

Analgesic/antipyretic: 10-15mg/kg/dose q4h up to a total of
60-80mg/kg/24h Max. dose: 4gm/24h
Anti-inflammatory: 60-100mg/kg/24h ÷ q6-8h
Kawasaki disease: 100mg/kg/24h PO ÷ QID during febrile phase
then decrease to 3-5mg/kg 24h PO qAM

Nursing Implications:

Do not use in children yr old with chicken pox or flu-like symptoms. Use with caution in GI disease. May cause GI upset, tinnitus. Therapeutic levels: 150-300mg/L.

BETHANECHOL

(Urecholine)

Implications:

Treatment of nonobstructive urinary retention and abdominal distention. Also effective in treatment of GE (gastroesophageal) reflux.

Administer:

Abdominal Distention/urinary retention:
    PO: 0.6mg/kg/24h ÷ q6-8h
    SC: 0.15-0.20mg/kg/24h ÷ q6-8h
GE Reflux:
    Children: 0.4mg/kg/24h ÷ QID (AC & HS) PO
    Adults: 10-50mg PO q6-12h

Nursing Implications:

Contraindicated in asthma, mechanical GI or GU obstruction, hyperthyroidism, seizure disorder. Can cause hypotension, nausea, abdominal cramps, and increased salivation. Do not give IM or IV.

BISACODYL

(Ducolax)

Indications:

Evacuation of the colon. Indicated in treatment of constipation associated with bed rest or spinal cord injury. Also used as prep for surgery or x-ray studies.

Administer:

Oral:
>   Child: 0.3mg/kg/24h or 5-10mg 6h prior to desired effect
>   Adult: 12yr: 5-15mg QD

Rectal:
>   <2yr: 5mg
>   2-11yr: 5-10mg
>   >11yr: 10mg

Nursing Implications:

Tablets should not be crushed or chewed. Do not give within one hour of milk or antacids. Can cause nausea and abdominal cramping. Oral dose effective in 6-10h. Rectal within 15-60min.

CALCITRIOL

(Rocaltrol)

Indications:

Most potent Vitamin D form available. Used most often in management of hypocalcemia in chronic renal failure. Promotes absorption of calcium from GI tract.

Administer:

Children: Range 0.01-0.05 mcg/kg/24h PO. Is titrated 0.005-0.01
mcg/kg/24h increments q4-8wk based on clinical response.
Adult: Initial: 0.25mcg/24h PO
Increment: 0.25mcg/24h PO q2-4wk

Nursing Implications:

Serum calcium and phosphorus levels must be monitored. Eating
foods high in calcium can lead to hypercalcemia. Can cause
weakness, headache, vomiting, constipation.

CAPTOPRIL

(Capoten)

Indications:

Management of hypertension. Also used in combination with other
drugs for treatment of congestive heart failure.

Administer:

Neonates: 0.1-0.4mg/kg/24h PO q6-8h
Infants: Initial dose: 0.15-0.3 mg /kg/dose titrated upward for
desired effect. Max. dose: 6mg/kg/24h ÷ QD-QID
Children: Initial dose: 0.5-1mg/kg/24h ÷ q8h titrated to minimal
effective dose. Max. dose: 6mg/kg/24h ÷ QD-QID
Adolescents & adults: Initial dose: 12-25mg/dose PO TID increased
weekly by 25mg/dose if necessary. Max. dose: 450mg/24h

Nursing Implications:

Should be given one hour prior to meals. Reaches peak 1-2 hours
after administration. Check baseline BP prior to administration.

CARBAMAZEPINE

(Tegretol)

Indications:

Anticonvulsant used to prevent tonic-clonic, mixed, and complex-partial seizures.

Administer:

< 6yr: Initial: 5-10mg/kg/24h PO ÷ BID
    Increment: q5-7 days up to 20mg/kg/24h PO
6-12yr: Initial: 10mg/kg/24h PO ÷ BID to max. of 100mg/dose
    BID
    Maintenance: 20-30mg/kg/24h po ÷ BID-QID
    Max. dose: 1000mg/24h
12yr: Initial: 200mg PO BID, Incremented at daily intervals
    Maintenance: 600-1200mg/24h PO ÷ BID-QID
    Max. dose: 12-15yr: 1000mg/24h, Adult: 1200mg/24h

Nursing Implications:

Therapeutic blood levels 4-12mg/L. Erythromycin, INH, Cimetidine, and Verapamil increase levels.

CEFACLOR

(Ceclor)

Indications:

Treatment of otitis media, respiratory, skin, bone and joint, and urinary tract infections.

Administer:

Infant and child: 40mg/kg/24h/PO ÷ q8h Max. dose: 2gm/24h
Adult: 250-500mg/dose PO q8h Max. dose: 4gm/24h

Nursing Implications:

Use with caution in children with penicillin sensitivity or impaired renal function. Safe use in infants mo not established.

CEFAZOLIN

(Ancef, Kefzol)

Indications:

Treatment of serious skin infections, urinary tract, bone and joint infections and septicemia. Also as prophylactic antibiotic for invasive procedures.

Administer:

Neonate: $\geq$2kg, $\geq$7 days old: 60mg/kg/24h $\div$ q8-12h IV/IM
Infant 1mo/children: 50-100mg/kg/24h $\div$ q6-8h IV/IM
Adult: 2-6gm/24h $\div$ q6-8h IV/IM
    Max. dose: 6gm/24h
IV dilution: Direct IV: Max. conc: 100mg/ml over 3-5 min.
    Intermittent infusion: 20mg/ml over 10-60 min.
Compatibility: D5, NS, LR

Nursing Implications:

Use with caution in children with penicillin sensitivity or impaired renal function.

CEFIXIME

(Suprax)

Indications:

Treatment of mild UTI's, otitis media, bronchitis, pharyngitis, or tonsillitis.

Administer:

Infant and child: 8mg/kg24h ÷ q12-24h PO Max. dose: 400mg/24h
Adult: 400mg/24h ÷ q12-24h PO

Nursing Implications:

Use with caution in children with penicillin sensitivity or impaired renal function. Can cause diarrhea, abdominal pain, nausea, headache.

CEFOTAXIME

(Claforan)

Indications:

Treatment of skin, bone, joint, urinary, gynecologic, respiratory, intra-abdominal infections. Septicemia and meningitis also.

Administer:

Infant and child: 100-200mg/kg/24h ÷ q12h IV/IM
        Meningitis: 200mg/kg/24h ÷ q6h IV/IM
Adults: 2-12gm/24h ÷ q4-8h IV/IM Max. dose: 12gm/24h
IV dilution: Direct IV: max. conc: 100-200mg/ml over 3-5 min.
        Intermittent infusion: 20-60mg/ml over 10-30 min.
Compatibility: D5, NS, LR

Nursing Implications:

Use with caution in penicillin sensitive children and with impaired renal function. Can cause neutropenia, thrombocytopenia.

CEFOXITIN

(Mefoxin)

Indications:

Treatment of skin, bone, joint, respiratory tract, urinary tract and gynecological infections.

Administer:

Infant and child: 80-160mg/kg/24h ÷ q4-6h IV/IM
Adult: 4-12gm/24h ÷ q6-8h IV/IM
    Max. dose: 12gm/24h
IV dilution: Direct IV: Max. conc: 100mg/ml over 3-5 min.
    Intermittent infusion: 10-40mg/ml over 10-60 min.
Compatibility: D5, NS, LR

Nursing Implications:

Use with caution with penicillin sensitive children and in impaired renal function.

CEFTAZIDIME

(Fortaz, and others)

Indications:

As in Cefoxitin plus inta-abdominal infections, septicemia, meningitis, and CF (Cystic Fibrosis)

Administer:

Infant and child: 90-150mg/kg/24h ÷ q8h IV/IM
Cystic Fibrosis: 150mg/kg/24h ÷ q8h IV/IM
Adult: 2-6gm/24h ÷ 8-12h IV/IM
    Max. dose: 6gm/24h

IV dilution: Direct IV: Max. conc: 180mg/ml over 3-5 min.
Intermittent infusion (preferred): 10-20mg/ml over   10-30 min.
Compatibility: D5, NS, LR

Nursing Implications:

Use with caution in penicillin sensitive children and with impaired renal function. Can cause neutropenia, thrombocytopenia.

CEFTRIAXONE

(Rocephin)

Indications:

See Ceftazidime. Plus gonococcal prophylaxis.

Administer:

Infant and child: 50-75mg/kg/24h ÷ q12-24h IV/IM
    Meningitis: 100mg/kg/24h ÷ q12h IV/IM
Adult: 1-4gm/24h ÷ q12-24h IV/IM
    Max. dose: 4gm/24h
Gonococcal prophylaxis: 125mg IM X 1 dose for children -kg
IV dilution: Direct IV: Max. Conc: 40mg/ml over 3-5 min.
    Intermittent infusion (preferred): 10-40mg/ml over   10-30 min.
Compatibility: D5, NS, LR

Nursing Implications:

Use with caution in penicillin sensitive children or impaired renal function. May cause jaundice.

CEFUROXIME, CEFUROXIME AXETIL

(Zinacef,IV/IM, Ceftin, PO)

Indications:

Same as other Cephalosporins. Not recommended for meningitis. PO form used to treat otitis media, pharyngitis, and tonsillitis.

Administer:

Infant and child: 75-100mg/kg/24h ÷ q8h IV/IM Max. dose: 6gm/24h

Adult: 750mg-1.5gm/dose q8h IV/IM Max. dose: 9gm/24h

PO: Children: 30mg/kg/24h ÷ BID

Otitis media: 40mg/kg/24h ÷ BID

IV dilution: Direct IV: Max. Conc: 94mg/ml over 3-5min.

Intermittent infusion (preferred): 1-30mg/ml over 15-60 min.

Compatibility: D5, NS, LR

Nursing Implications:

Use with caution in penicillin sensitive children or impaired renal function. May cause thrombophlebitis at infusion site.

CEPHALEXIN

(Keflex)

Indications:

Same as other Cephalosporins. Not recommended for meningitis. PO form used to treat otitis media, pharyngitis, and tonsillitis.

Administer:

Infant and child: 25-50mg/kg/24h PO ÷ q6-12h

Adult: 1-4gm/24h PO ÷ q6-12h

Max. dose: 4gm/24h

Nursing Implications:

Use with caution in penicillin sensitive children and impaired renal function. Can cause GI disturbance. Give with food or milk to decrease GI irritation. Safety and effectiveness in children less than one month has not been established.

CHLORAL HYDRATE

(Noctec)

Indications:

Short-term sedative and hypnotic, preop sedation.

Administer:

Children:
    Sedative: 5-15mg/kg/dose q8h PO/PR
    Procedure: 25-100mg/kg/dose PO/PR Max: 2gm/dose
    Hypnotic: 50-75mg/kg/dose PO/PR Max: 1gm/dose, 2gm/24h
Adult:
    Sedative: 250mg/dose TID PO/PR
    Hypnotic: 500-1000mg/dose PO/PR Max: 2gm/24h

Nursing Implications:

Irritating to mucous membranes. Can cause GI irritation, paradoxical excitement, hypotension, heart and respiratory depression. Can accumulate with repeated use. Do not use in children with liver or renal impairment. Use caution in children with heart disease or on Furosemide or anticoagulants.

CHLORAMPHENICOL

(Chloromycetin)

Indications:

Treatment of skin and soft tissue, intra-abdominal, CNS infections, and bacteremia. Topical, ophthalmic for local management of superficial infections.

Administer:

Ophthalmic: 1-2gtts or ribbon of ointment in each eye q3-6h
Topical: Apply to affected area TID-QID
Loading dose (all ages): 20mg/kg IV/PO
Maintenance (all ages): 50-100mg/kg/24h IV/PO ÷ q6h
    Max. dose: 4gm/24h
IV dilution: Intermittent infusion: 20-100mg/ml over 30-60 min.
    DO NOT GIVE DIRECT IV.
Compatibility: D5, NS, LR

Nursing Implications:

Monitor blood levels. Can cause marrow suppression, "Gray Baby Syndrome." Therapeutic levels: 15-25mg/L, for meningitis: 10-20mg/L. PO doses achieve higher levels than IV doses.

CIMETIDINE

(Tagamet)

Indications:

Treatment and prophylaxis of duodenal ulcers. Treatment of benign gastric ulcers. Management of GE reflux and to inhibit gastric acid secretion.

Administer:

Infants: 10-20mg/kg/24h PO/IV ÷ q6h

Children: 20-40mg/kg/24h PO/IV ÷ q6h

Adult: 300mg/dose QID, 400mg/dose BID, or 800mg/dose QHS
PO/IV/IM
Ulcer prophylaxis: 400-800mg QHS PO: Max. dose:
2400mg/24h

IV dilution: Max. conc: 25mg/ml over 15-30 min.
DO NOT GIVE IV PUSH.

Nursing Implications:

Use with caution in all patients. Rapid IV administration can cause
hypotension, arrhythmias, cardiac arrest. Can cause confusion.

CLINDAMYCIN

(Cleocin)

Indications:

Treatment of skin, respiratory tract, inta-abdominal, and
gynecologic infections; septicemia and osteomyelitis.

Administer:

Term <1mo: 20-40mg/kg/24h ÷ q6h IV/IM

Children: 20-30mg/kg/24h ÷ q6h PO
25-40mg/kg/24h ÷ q6-8h IV/IM

Adult: 150-450mg/dose q6-8h PO
600-3600mg/24h ÷ q6-12h IV/IM
Max. dose: 4.8gm/24h IV/IM; 1.8gm/24h PO

IV dilution: Max. conc: 18mg/ml
Usual 6-12mg/ml over 10-60 min.
Do not exceed 30mg/min.

Compatibility: D5, NS, LR

Nursing Implications:

Contraindicated in liver impairment and diarrhea. Can cause diarrhea, rash. Rapid infusion can cause cardiac arrest.

CODEINE

(Many brands)

Indications:

Mild to moderate pain. Antitussive in smaller doses.

Administer:

Analgesic:
    Children: 0.5-1.0mg/kg/dose q4-6h IM,SC,PO
        Max: 60mg/dose
    Adult: 30-60mg/dose q4-6h IM,SC,PO
    Tylenol with Codeine:
        Elixir contains Acetaminophen 120mg and codeine 12mg/5ml
        Tablets with codeine all contain 300mg acetaminophen/tab
        Tylenol #1: 7.5mg codeine
        Tylenol #2: 15mg codeine
        Tylenol #3: 30mg codeine
        Tylenol #4: 60mg codeine
Antitussive: All doses PRN
    Children(2-6yr): 2.5-5.0mg/dose q4-6h PO
        Max. dose: 30mg/24h
    Children(6-12yr): 5-10mg/dose q4-6h
        Max. dose: 60mg/24h
    Adults: 15-30mg/dose q4-6h
        Max. dose: 120mg/24h

Nursing Implications:

Can cause CNS and respiratory depression, constipation, cramping. For pain effects use with acetaminophen.

CO-TRIMOXAZOLE

(Bactrim, Septra)

Indications:

Treatment of bronchitis, shigella, otitis media, pneumocystis carinii pneumonia (PCP), UTI's, and diarrhea. Also used as suppression therapy in chronic UTI's and to prevent PCP in children with HIV infection.

Administer:

Doses based on TMP component:
Minor infections:
    Child: 8-10mg/kg/24h ÷ q12h IV/PO
    Adult(40kg): 160mg/dose q12h
UTI Prophylaxis: 2mg/kg/24h QD
Severe infections & PCP: 20mg/kg/24h ÷ q6-8h IV/PO
PCP Prophylaxis: 5-10mg/kg/24h ÷ q12 3 consecutive days/wk
    Max. dose: 320mg/24h
IV dilution: 1mg/15ml over 60-90min
    DO NOT GIVE IV PUSH
Compatibility: D5

Nursing Implications:

Use cautiously with impaired renal or liver function. Not recommended in infants mo. May cause blood dyscrasias.

DIGOXIN

(Lanoxin)

Implications:

Treatment of CHF, to slow the heart rate in atrial fibrillation and flutter. To end paroxysmal atrial tachycardia. Increases the force of myocardial contraction, decreases conduction through the SA and AV node. Increases cardiac output.

Administer:

Maintenance doses:

Neonate:	8-10mcg/kg/24h PO BID	
	6-10mcg/kg/24h IV/IM BID	
Children <2yr:		10-12mcg/kg/24h PO BID
	7.5-9mcg/kg/24h IV/IM BID	
2-10yr:	8-10mcg/kg/24h PO BID	
	6-8mcg/kg/24h IV/IM BID	
>10yr:	125-250mcg/24h QD PO/IV/IM	

IV dilution: Undiluted or diluted at least 4 fold over 5 min.
    Max. conc: Child: 100mcg/ml, Adult: 250mcg/ml
Compatibility: D5,NS,SW

Nursing Implications:

Check apical pulse for one full minute before administration. Hold dose and check with doctor if HR Z-100 BPM for an infant, 70 BPM for a child, and 60 BPM for an adult or according to hospital policy. IV dose should be double checked before administering. Less than 4-fold dilution can cause precipitation. Therapeutic levels: 0.8-2.0mcg/ml. Most common side effects in infants and children are nausea and vomiting.

DIPHENHYDRAMINE

(Benadryl)

Indications:

Treatment of allergic symptoms caused by histamine release such as nasal allergies, anaphylaxis.

Administer:

Children: 5mg/kg/24h ÷ q6h PO/IV/IM Max. dose: 300mg/24h
Adult: 10-50mg/dose q6-8h PO/IV/IM Max. dose: 400mg/24h
Anaphylaxis: 1-2mg/kg/IV
IV dilution: Max. conc: 50mg/ml over 5 min
    Intermittent infusion: 10-50mg/ml over 15 min.
Compatibility: D5, NS, LR

Nursing Implications:

Contraindicated in asthma. Use cautiously in liver impairment. Can cause drowsiness, dizziness, and dry mouth.

DOCUSATE SODIUM

(Colace)

Indications:

Stool softener used to prevent constipation.

Administer:

<3yr: 10-40mg/24h ÷ QD-QID PO
3-6yr: 20-60mg/24h ÷ QD-QID PO
6-12yr: 40-120mg/24h ÷ QD-QID PO
>12yr: 50-500mg/24h ÷ QD-QID PO

Nursing Implications:

Prolonged use leads to dependence. Oral dose may take 1-3 days of therapy to be effective. Oral solution better tolerated with milk or fruit juice.

ERYTHROMYCIN

(Many different preparations)

Indications:

PO/IV: Treatment of upper and lower respiratory tract infections, skin infections, pertussis, diphtheria, rheumatic fever, and chlamydia. Topical: acne. Ophthalmic: superficial infections.

Administer:

PO: Neonate ≤ 7 days: 20mg/kg/24h ÷ q12h
             > 7 days: 30mg/kg/24h ÷ q8h
    Children: 30-50mg/kg/24h ÷ q6-8h Max. dose: 2gm/24h
    Adults: 1-4gm/24h ÷ q6h Max. dose: 4gm/24h
IV: Children: 20-50mg/kg/24h ÷ q6h
    Adults: 15-20mg/kg/24h ÷ q6h Max. dose: 4gm/24h
IV dilution: Max. conc: 5mg/ml
               Usual 1-2.5mg/ml over 20-60 min.
               DO NOT GIVE IV PUSH
Compatibility: D5, NS, LR

Nursing Implications:

Nausea, vomiting, abdominal cramps common. Give after meals. Use with caution in liver disease. Can increase digoxin, theophylline, carbamazapine, cyclosporine, and methylpredniso-lone levels.

ERYTHROMYCIN ETHYLSUCCINATE AND ACETYL SULFISOXAZOLE

(Pediazole)

Indications:

Otitis media.

Administer:

50mg/kg/24h erythromycin and 150mg/kg/24h of sulfa ÷ q6h PO
or 1.25ml/kg/24h ÷ q6h PO Max. dose: 6gm sulfisoxazole/24h

Nursing Implications:

Same as erythromycin. Not recommended in infants mo.

FOLIC ACID

(Folate, Folvite)

Indications:

To stimulate production of red blood cells, white blood cells and platelets.

Administer:

Maintenance: PO/IV/IM/SC
< 1yr:	30-45mcg/24h
1-3yr:	100mcg/24h
4-6yr:	200mcg/24h
7-10yr:	300mcg/24h
11-adult:	400mcg/24h

Nursing Implications:

Urine may appear more yellow.

FUROSEMIDE

(Lasix)

Indications:

Management of edema from CHF.

Administer:

PO: Infants & children: 2mg/kg/dose q6-8h prn: May increase by
1-2mg/kg/dose to max of 6mg/kg/24h

Adult: 20-80mg/24h QD or BID up to 600mg/24h

IV: Infants & children: 1mg/kg/dose q6-12h prn, may increase by
1mg./kg/dose to max of 6mg/kg/24h

Adult: 20-80mg/dose Max single dose: 6mg/kg

IV dose may also be given IM

IV dilution: 10mg/ml over 1-2 min. Max 0.5mg/kg/min. or
4mg/min

Compatibility: D5, NS, LR

Nursing Implications:

Use cautiously in liver disease. May cause hypokalemia. Observe
for dehydration.

GENTAMYCIN

(Garamycin)

Indications:

Treatment of serious gram negative bacillary infections of the
respiratory tract, skin, abdomen, urinary tract; and endocarditis and
septicemia.

Administer:

Children: 6-7.5mg/kg/24h ÷ q8h IV/IM

Adult: 3-5mg/kg/24h ÷ q8h IV/IM
     Max. dose: 300mg/24h
IV dilution: 1mg/ml, max conc: 2mg/ml over 30-60 min
     DO NOT GIVE IV PUSH
Compatibility: D5, NS

Nursing Implications:

Ototoxic and nephrotoxic. Monitor levels. Therapeutic levels: Peak: 6-10mg/L; Trough: mg/L.

HYDROXYZINE

(Atarax, Vistaril)

Indications:

Treatment of anxiety, pre-op sedation, antiemetic, and antipruritic.

Administer:

PO: Children: 2mg/kg/24h ÷ q6h
     Adult: 25-100mg/dose TID-QID
IM: Children: 0.5-1.0mg/kg/dose q4-6h PRN
     Adult: 25-100mg/dose q4-6h PRN
               Max. dose: 600mg/24h
               NEVER GIVE IV

Nursing Implications:

Potentiates barbiturates and meperidine. Can cause dry mouth and drowsiness.

IBUPROFEN

(Motrin, Advil, and others)

Indications:

Management of inflammatory disorders such as juvenile rheumatoid arthritis(JRA), and as an analgesic for mild to moderate pain. Also used as antipyretic.

Administer:

Children:
    Antipyretic: 20mg/kg/24h ÷ q8h PO
    JRA: 20-40mg/kg/24h ÷ q6-8h PO
        Max. dose: 40mg/kg/24h
Adult:
    Inflammatory disease: 400-800mg/dose q6-8h
    Pain/fever: 200-400mg/dose q4-6h
        Max. dose: 3.2gm/24h

Nursing Implications:

Use with caution with liver and renal impairment. Can cause nausea, vomiting. GI problems can be lessened by administration with milk.

IRON

(Many preparations)

Indications:

Prevention and treatment of iron deficiency anemia.

Administer:

Treatment: 3-6mg elemental Fe/kg/24h ÷ TID PO
Prevention:
    Premature: 2mg elemental Fe/kg/24h

Term & children: 1-2mg elemental Fe/kg/24h
        Max. dose: 15mg elemental Fe/24h
    Adult: 100mg elemental Fe/24h PO ÷ QD-BID

Nursing Implications:

Liquid preparations stain teeth. Use dropper or straw to administer. Less GI irritation if given after meals. May cause constipation, dark stools, nausea and epigastric pain.

KANAMYCIN

(Kantrex)

Indications:

Treatment of gram negative bacillary and staphylococcal infections of bone, respiratory tract, skin, abdomen, and complicated UTI's; also endocarditis and septicemia.

Administer:

Infants & children: 15-30mg/kg/24h ÷ q8-12h IV/IM
                Max. dose: 1.5gm/24h
Adult: 15mg/kg/24h ÷ q8-12h IV/IM
                Max. dose: 1.5gm/24h
IV dilution: Max. conc: 5mg/ml
                Usual 2.5mg/ml over 30 min.
                DO NOT GIVE IV PUSH
Compatibility: D5, NS, LR

Nursing Implications:

Ototoxic, retinal toxic, and nephrotoxic. Therapeutic levels: Peak: 15-30mg/L; Trough: -10mg/L.

MEPERIDINE

(Demerol and others)

Indications:

Narcotic used in management of moderate to severe pain. Also used as preop sedation.

Administer:

PO/IV/IM/SC
Children: 1.0-1.5mg/kg/dose q3-4h PRN Max. dose: 100mg
Adult: 50-100mg/dose q3-4h PRN
IV dilution: give undiluted or .6-10mg/ml direct IV over 5 min.
   Infusion: 0.3-1.5mg/kg/hr
Compatibility: D5, NS, LR

Nursing Implications:

Lower dose if given IV. Can cause nausea, vomiting, respiratory depression, constipation and lethargy. Continued use decreases effects. Not recommended for chronic use.

METHICILLIN

(Staphcillin)

Indications:

Treatment of respiratory tract, skin, bone, joint, urinary tract infections, and endocarditis, septicemia, and meningitis due to susceptible strains of penicillinase-producing staphylococci.

Administer:

Neonates > 1wk: 25-50mg/kg/dose q6h IV/IM
Infants 1mo & children: 100-400mg/kg/24h ÷ q4-6h IV/IM

Adult: 4-12gm/24h ÷ q4-6h IV/IM
     Max. dose: 12gm/24h
IV dilution: 2-20mg/ml over 15-30 min.
Compatibility: D5,NS,LR

Nursing Implications:

Can cause hematuria, reversible bone marrow depression, rash, and phlebitis at IV site. Dose decreased in renal impairment.

METHYLPREDNISOLONE

(Medrol, Solu-medrol, and others)

Indications:

Management of chronic inflammatory, allergic, hematologic, neoplastic, and autoimmune diseases.

Administer:

Anti-inflammatory/immunosuppressive:
     0.16-0.8mg/kg/24h PO/IV/IM ÷ q6-12h
Status asthmaticus:
     Child:
          Loading: 1-2mg/kg/dose IV X 1
          Maintenance: 2mg/kg/24h ÷ q6h IV
     Adult: 10-250mg/dose q4-6h IV/IM
IV dilution: Undiluted for push. Max. conc: 62.5mg/ml over 3-5min
     Infusion: 2.5mg/ml over 20-60 min.
Compatibility: D5, NS

Nursing Implications:

Monitor blood pressure with IV infusion. Should never be abruptly discontinued.

MORPHINE

(various names)

Indications:

Management of severe pain. Effective with painful sickle cell crisis and cyanotic spells associated with tetralogy.

Administer:

Analgesia/tetralogy spells:
>   Neonates: 0.05-0.2mg/kg/dose Slow IV/IM/SC q4h
>   Child: 0.1-0.2mg/kg/dose IV/IM/SC q2-4h PRN
>   Max. dose: 15mg/dose
>   Adult:
>   PO: 10-30mg q4h PRN
>   IV: 2-15mg/dose q2-6h PRN

Continuous IV: 0.025-2mg/kg/hr begin at lower dose and titrated to effect
>   Direct IV: undiluted 1-5mg/ml over 4-5 min.

Compatibility: D5

Nursing Implications:

Can cause hypotension, constipation. Assess for sedation and respiratory depression.

NAFCILLIN

(Unipen, Nafcil)

Indications:

Treatment of penicillinase-producing staphylococci infections of the respiratory tract, bone, joints, skin, and urinary tract. Also endocarditis, septicemia, and meningitis.

Administer:

Neonate >7 days: 75mg/kg/24h ÷ q6h IV/IM
Infants & children:
    PO: 50-100mg/kg/24h ÷ q6h
    IM: 100-200mg/kg/24h ÷ q12h
    IV: 100-200mg/kg/24h ÷ q6h
Adult:
    PO: 250-1000mg q4-6h
    IV/IM: 500-2000mg q4-6h
    Max. dose: 12gm/24h
IV dilution: 2-40mg/ml over 60 min.
Compatibility: D5, NS, LR

Nursing Implications:

High incidence of phlebitis with IV route. Decrease rate and/or concentration for vein irritation. Sodium bicarb may be added to IV dilution to buffer effects. Warm or cold compresses at IV site may help to decrease pain during infusion.

NITROFURANTOIN

(Furadantin, Macrodantin)

Indications:

Treatment of urinary tract infections and for chronic suppression therapy of urinary tract infections.

Administer:

Children >1mo:
    Treatment: 5-7mg/kg/24h ÷ q6h PO
    Prophylaxis: 1-3mg/kg q HS PO
        Max. dose: 400mg/24h
Adult:
    Treatment: 50-100mg/dose q6h PO

Prophylaxis: 50-100mg PO q HS

Nursing Implications:

Can cause nausea, vomiting, headache. Contraindicated in severe renal disease, G6PD deficiency, and infants 1mo. Give with food or milk.

NYSTATIN

(Mycostatin, Nilstat, and others)

Indications:

PO, topical, vaginal treatment of candida infections.

Administer:

Oral:
> Pre-term infants: 0.5ml (50,000u) to each side of the mouth QID
> Term infants: 1ml (100,000u) to each side of the mouth QID
> Children & adult: 4-6ml (400,000-600,000u) swish and swallow QID

Vaginal: 1 Tab q HS X 10 days

Topical: Apply to affected area BID-QID

Nursing Implications:

May need to paint on lesions in mouth with Q-tip with infants. Can cause GI effects. Must continue to treat until 48-72h after lesions are gone.

PENICILLIN G

(Potassium and sodium preparations)

Indications:

Treatment of infections including: Pneumococcal pneumonia, streptococcal pharyngitis, syphilis, and gonorrhea. Also used to treat lyme disease and prevent rheumatic fever.

Administer:

Neonate: > 7days > 2kg: 100,000-200,000u/kg/24h ÷ q6h IV/IM
Congenital syphilis:

    > 7 days: 100,000u/kg/24h ÷ q12h IV/IM
    7-28 days: 150,000u/kg/24h ÷ q8h IV/IM
    28 days: 200,000u/kg/24h ÷ q6h IV/IM
    Treat for 10-14 days

Children:

    IV/IM: 100,000-400,000u/kg/24h ÷ q4-6h
       Max. dose: 24 million units/24h
    PO: 40,000-80,000u/kg/24h ÷ q6-8h or 25-50mg/kg/24h ÷
       q6-8h

Adult:

    IV/IM: 2-24 million units/24h ÷ q4-6h
    PO: 200,000-800,000u/dose q6-8h or 125-500mg/dose q6-8h
IV dilution: 100,000-500,000u/ml over 15-30 min.
Compatibility: D5, NS, LR

Nursing Implications:

Dose adjustment in renal impairment. Oral should be taken 1-2 hours before or 2 hours after meals. Can cause anaphylaxis, hemolytic anemia.

PENICILLIN G

Benzathine preparations
(Bicillin L-A)

Indications:

Same as Penicillin G potassium/sodium preparations.

Administer:

Syphilis, early acquired:
    Infants & children: 50,000u/kg X 1 dose IM
        Max. dose: 2.4 million units
    Adult: 1.2 million units X 1 IM
Syphilis for > 1 yr:
    Infants & children: 50,000u/kg IM q wk X 3 doses
        Max. dose: 2.4 million u/dose
    Adult: 2.4 million u/dose IM q wk X 3 doses
Group A streptococci:
    Infants & children: 50,000u/kg X 1 dose IM
        Max. dose: 1.2 million u/dose
    Adult: 1.2 million units X 1 dose IM
Rheumatic fever prophylaxis:
    Infants & children: 25,000u/kg IM q3-4wk
        Max. dose: 1.2 million u/dose
    Adult: 1.2 million units IM q3-4wk or 600,000u IM q2wk

Nursing Implications:

Do not give IV.

PENICILLIN G

Procaine preparations
(Duricillin A.S.,Crysticillin A.S.)

Indications:

Same as Penicillin G potassium/sodium

Administer:

Infants & children: 25,000-50,000u/kg/24h ÷ q12-24 h IM
    Max. dose: 4.8 million u/24h
Adult: 0.6-4.8 million u/24h ÷ q12-24h IM
Congenital syphilis: 50,000u/kg/24h ÷ q12-24h IM X 10-14 days
Syphilis: 12yr-adult: 600,000u QD IM X 8-15 days

Nursing Implications:

Do not give IV. May cause pain at IM injection site.

PENICILLIN V POTASSIUM

(Pen Vee K, V-cillin K)

Indications:

Same as other penicillins.

Administer:

Children: 25-50mg/kg/24h ÷ q6h PO Max. dose: 3gm/24h
Adult: 250-500mg/dose PO q6h
Secondary Rheumatic fever/Pneumococcal prophylaxis:
    ≤5 yrs: 125mg PO BID
    > 5 yrs: 250mg PO BID

Nursing Implications:

Better GI absorbed than Penicillin G. Must be taken 1 hour before or 2 hours after meals.

PHENOBARBITAL

(Luminal)

Indications:

Used as anticonvulsant in grand mal, partial, and febrile seizures. Also for sedation.

Administer:

Sedation:
> Children: 6mg/kg/24h PO ÷ TID
> Adult: 30-120mg/24h PO ÷ BID-TID

Status epilepticus:
> Loading dose IV:
>> Neonate: 15-20mg/kg in single or divided dose
>> Infants/children/adult: 15-18mg/kg in single or divided dose, increased 5mg/kg q15-30 min to max: 30mg/kg

> Maintenance dose PO/IV:
>> Neonate: 3-4mg/kg/24h ÷ QD-BID
>> Infants: 5-6mg/kg/24h ÷ QD-BID
>> 1-5yr:6-8mg/kg/24h ÷ QD-BID
>> 6-12yr: 4-6mg/kg/24h ÷ QD-BID
>> >12yr:1-3mg/kg/24h ÷ QD-BID
>> Max. dose: 1-2gm

IV dilution: Give undiluted or dilute with equal volume
> Direct IV: 1mg/min
> Infusion: over 20-30 min.

Compatibility: D5, NS, LR

Nursing Implications:

IV route usually for emergency use only. May cause respiratory arrest or hypotension. Can cause hyperactivity, irritability, insomnia as paradoxical reaction in children. Therapeutic levels: 15-40mg/L.

PHENYTOIN

(Dilantin)

Indications:

Treatment and prevention of grand mal seizures and complex partial seizures.

Administer:

Maintenance for seizure disorders:
Neonates: 5-8mg/kg/24h PO/IV ÷ q8-12h
Infants & children: start 5mg/kg/24h ÷ QD-q12h PO/IV
Usual ranges:
    6mo-3yr: 8-10mg/kg/24h
    4-6yr: 7.5-9mg/kg/24h
    7-9yr: 7-8mg/kg/24h
    10-16yr: 6-7mg/kg/24h
    all divided q8-12h
IV dilution: give undiluted or dilute with normal saline 1-10mg/ml to max: 50mg/ml. Direct IV not to exceed 0.5mg/kg/min. Flush with normal saline. Diluted solutions mist be administered within one hour.
Compatibility: NS only

Nursing Implications:

Crystallizes with dextrose. Sometimes also used antiarrhythmic. Assess for irritation and necrosis with IV use. Therapeutic levels for seizure disorders: 10-20mg/L.

PIPERACILLIN

(Pipracil)

Indications:

Treatment of serious infections of skin, bone, joint, respiratory tract, and urinary tract. Also intra-abdominal and gynecologic infections. Often used for respiratory infections in children with cystic fibrosis(CF).

Administer:

Children > 12yr with CF: 300-600mg/kg/24h ÷ q4-6h IV/deepIM
Others: 200-300mg/kg/24h ÷ q4-6h IV/deepIM
    Max. dose: 24gm/24h
Adult: 3-4gm/dose IV q4-6h or 2-3gm/dose IM q6-12h
    Max. dose: 24gm/24h
IV dilution: 10-20mg/ml over 30-60 min. Max. conc: 200-300mg/ml
Compatibility: D5, NS, LR

Nursing Implications:

Reactions similar to penicillins. Assess IV site for irritation and phlebitis.

POTASSIUM CHLORIDE

(KCl supplements)

Indications:

To correct or prevent potassium imbalance.

Administer:

Infants & children: 2-3mEq/kg/24h to Max. of 40mEq/24h
Adult: 40-80mEq/24h

IV dilution: Max. peripheral IV solution concentration: 40mEq/L
    Max. infusion rate: 0.5-1mEq/kg/hr
    DO NOT GIVE IV PUSH
Compatibility: D5, NS, LR

Nursing Implications:

Rapid IV infusion can cause arrhythmias. Monitor potassium levels.

PREDNISONE

(Deltasone)

Indications:

Used systemically and locally in a wide range of diseases including:
inflammatory, allergic, hematologic, neoplastic, and autoimmune.

Administer:

Anti-inflammatory/immunosuppressive:
    0.5-2mg/kg/24h ÷ q6-12h PO
Asthma:
    Acute: 0.5-2mg/kg/24h up to 20-40mg/24h PO X 3-5days
    Chronic: 5-10mg/dose QD or 10-30mg QOD
Nephrotic Syndrome:
    Initial: 2mg/kg/24h ÷ TID-QID PO Max. dose: 80mg/24h X
        28 days. Can increase to 4mg/kg/dose QOD X another 28
        days. Max. dose: 120mg/24h
    Maintenance: 2mg/kg/dose QOD X 28 days

Nursing Implications:

Doses must be tapered gradually to discontinue.

PROMETHAZINE

(Phenergan)

Indications:

Preop sedation, treatment and prevention of nausea and vomiting.

Administer:

Sedation: 0.5-1.1mg/kg/dose PO/PR/IV/IM
Nausea & vomiting:
    Children: 0.25-0.5mg/kg/dose PO/PR/IV/IM q4-6h PRN
    Adult: 12.5-25mg q4-6h PRN
IV dilution: As desired. Max. conc: 25mg/ml no faster than
    25mg/min.
Compatibility: D5, NS, LR

Nursing Implications:

Observe for excessive sedation. Monitor BP, pulse and respirations
with IV use.

RANITIDINE

(Zantac)

Indications:

Treatment and prevention of duodenal ulcers. Management of GE
reflux.

Administer:

Children:	PO: 2-4mg/kg/24h ÷ q12h
	IV: 1-2mg/kg/24h ÷ q6-8h
Adult:	PO: 150mg BID or 300mg QHS
	IV: 50mg q6-8h
IV dilution:	Max. conc: 2.5mg/ml over 5 min.
	Infusion: 0.5-2.5mg/ml over 15-20 min.

Compatibility: D5, NS, LR

Nursing Implications:

Rapid infusion can cause bradycardia, tachycardia, or PVC's. Can be added to TPN. Can cause headache, GI disturbances, malaise, sedation. May also increase theophylline levels.

RIFAMPIN

(Rimactane)

Indications:

Management of active tuberculosis, eliminate carriers of meningococcal disease, prophylaxis for H-Influenza type B infection.

Administer:

Children: 10-20mg/kg/24h IV/PO ÷ q12-24h
TB: 10-20mg/kg/dose up to Max. of 600mg/dose PO QD or twice
    a week
Meningitis prophylaxis:
    0-1mo: 10mg/kg/24h ÷ q12h X 2 days
    > 1mo: 20mg/kg/24h to max of 600mg/dose ÷ q12 h PO X 2
    days
H-Flu: 0-1mo: 10mg/kg/24h PO QD x 4 days
    > 1mo: 20mg/kg/24h PO Max. of 600mg/dose/24h X 4 days
IV dilution: Max. conc: 6mg/ml
    Usual: 1-2mg/ml over 30-60 min. to max. of 3 hours
Compatibility: D5

Nursing Implications:

Causes red discoloration of body fluids. Give 1 hour before or 2 hours after meals. May cause GI irritation, headache, ataxia, fever and blood dyscrasias.

SULFISOXAZOLE

(Gantisin)

Indications:

Treatment of urinary tract infections.

Administer:

Children > 2mo:
    Initial: 75mg/kg/dose PO X 1
    Maintenance: 150mg/kg/24h ÷ q4-6h PO
        Max. dose: 6gm/24h
Adult:
    Loading: 2-4gm X 1
    Maintenance: 4-8gm/24h ÷ q4-6h PO
        Max. dose: 8gm/24h

Nursing Implications:

Do not use in infants mo of age. Maintain adequate fluid intake.

THEOPHYLLINE

(Many brands)

Indications:

Same as aminophylline.

Administer:

Maintenance: PO
    0-2mo: 3-6mg/kg/24h ÷ q8h
    2-6mo: 6-15mg/kg/24h ÷ q6h
    6-12mo: 15-22mg/kg/24h ÷ q4-6h
    1-9yr: 22mg/kg/24h ÷ q4-6h
    10-16yr: 18mg/kg/24h ÷ q6h

Adult: 13mg/kg/24h ÷ q6h
Max. dose: 900mg/24h

Nursing Implications:

Must check levels. Therapeutic for bronchospasm: 10-20mg/L. For apnea: 7-13mg/L. Most common side effects are same as Aminophylline.

TICARCILLIN

(Ticar)

Indications:

Treatment of serious infections of skin, bone, joints, respiratory tract, and urinary tract; and septicemia, inta-abdominal and gynecologic infections.

Administer:

Neonates > 7 days > 2 kg: 300mg/kg/24h ÷ q8h IV
Children & adult: 200-300mg/kg/24h ÷ q4-6h IV/IM
    Max. dose: 24-30gm/24h
Uncomplicated UTI:
    Children: 50-100mg/kg/24h ÷ q6-8h IV/IM
    Adult: 1gm q6h IV/IM
        Max. IM dose: 2gm/injection
CF: 300-600mg/kg/24h ÷ q4-6h IV/IM
IV dilution: 10-100mg/ml over 30-120 min.
Compatibility: D5, NS, LR

Nursing Implications:

May cause decreased platelet aggregation, hypocalcemia.

TICARCILLIN/CLAVULANATE

(Timentin)

Indications:

Same as ticarcillin except has beta-lactamase inhibitor that broadens spectrum.

Administer:

Same as ticarcillin except Max. dose: 18-20gm/24h

Nursing Implications:

Same as ticarcillin.

TOBRAMYCIN

(Tobrex)

Indications:

Treatment of serious gram negative infections and staphylococcal infections when penicillin is contraindicated or gentamycin resistance has occurred.

Administer:

Children: 6-7.5mg/kg/24h ÷ q8h IV/IM
Adult: 3-5mg/kg/24h ÷ q8h IV/IM
IV dilution: 1mg/ml to max. conc of 2mg/ml over 30-60 min.
    DO NOT GIVE IV PUSH
Compatibility: D5, NS
Ophthalmic: ointment: BID-TID. solution: 1-2 drops q4h

Nursing Implications:

Therapeutic levels: Peak: 6-10mg/L. Trough: mg/L. Can cause ototoxicity, nephrotoxicity. Children with CF or neutropenia may need higher doses.

VALPROIC ACID

(Depakane)

Indications:

Treatment of simple and complex absence seizures.

Administer:

Initial: 10-15mg/kg/24h ÷ QD-TID PO can be incrementally increased at weekly intervals to maintenance dose.
Maintenance: 30-60mg/kg/24h ÷ QD-TID PO
    Max. dose: 60mg/kg/24h

Nursing Implications:

Can cause GI, blood, CNS, and liver toxicity; weight gain, and transient alopecia. Do not give with carbonated beverages. Therapeutic levels: 50-100mg/L.

VANCOMYCIN

(Vancocin)

Indications:

Treatment of life-threatening infections when less toxic antibiotics are contraindicated. Especially useful in treating staphylococcal infections.

Administer:

Infants & children:
    CNS: 15mg/kg/dose q8h IV
    Other: 10mg/kg/dose q8h IV
Adult: 2gm/24h ÷ q6-12h IV
IV dilution: 2.5-5mg/ml over 60 min.
Compatibility: D5, NS, LR

Nursing Implications:

"Red man syndrome" with too rapid infusion. (Red flushing of neck and head). Ototoxic and nephrotoxic. Therapeutic levels: Peak: 25-40mg/L. Trough: mg/L.

IV FLUID DILUTION AND RATE CALCULATIONS

To determine proper dilution:
Recommended dilution of a particular drug is 10mg/ml.
Patient's dose is 500mg IV q6h.
To determine the amount of fluid to dilute it in:

$$\frac{10mg}{1ml} = \frac{500mg}{x\ ml} \qquad \text{Cross multiply}$$

$$10x = 500$$
$$x = 50 \text{ ml. So you will dilute 500mg}$$
in 50mls to get the proper
concentration of 10mg/ml.

To determine the proper rate:

$$\frac{\text{Vol. to be infused} \times \text{the drip factor}}{\text{time in minutes}} = \text{drops(gtts)/minute}$$

Ex. We want to dilute the above drug in 50mls. and give over 30 minutes. The drip factor in pedi is usually 60 because of the use of microdrips.

$$\frac{20ml \times 60}{30min.} = 40gtts/min \text{ or with drip factor of 60, is also}$$
40ml/hour.

SAFE DRUG CALCULATIONS

Determine child's weight in kg.
Ex. Child weighs 22 pounds. 22 pounds ÷ 2.2 pounds/kg = 10 kg.

Recommended safe dose is 200-400mg/kg/24h given q6h.
Multiply 200mg × 10kg and 400mg × 10kg to get a safe range for the 24h. Safe range is 2000mg-4000mg/24h. Divide by 4 to get the safe range for each dose given q6h. Safe dose range is 500mg-1000mg/dose.

The above drug comes in a solution of 1000mg/ml. We want to give a dose of 500mg. To calculate amount to draw up:

$$\frac{1000mg}{1ml} = \frac{500mg}{x\ ml} \quad \text{Cross multiply}$$

$$1000\ x = 500$$

$$x = .5\ ml$$

PREPARATION FOR ADMINISTRATION

GENERAL GUIDELINES

Start with clean area.

Obtain proper drug, proper strength.

Assemble needed equipment.

Draw-up medication or check unit dose.

Make sure you have everything needed before entering patient's room. i.e., alcohol swab, bandaid, proper needle for IV system, label, nipple, syringe, cup, drink, etc.

Take med sheet or card to compare to patients ID band.

Know how patient has taken and tolerated medications before. ie. Can he swallow pills, can he tolerate the volume?

NO meds in playroom. This is a safe area. Take child out of the playroom to administer any medication.

Be truthful, let the child know what to expect. Explain child's and parent's roles. Try not to let the parent threaten the child. Encourage parents to comfort only.

Infants	Need TLC before and after.
Toddlers	Need immediate preparation. Don't offer unreal choices. Allow parent to help with oral meds.
Pre-school	Need to know what they are expected to do. Let them handle the equipment. Bandaid very important for body integrity.
School-age	Need an explanation of their role and choices when possible. Longer preparation time is needed for invasive procedures.
Adolescent	Generally want more information. Privacy is important. Preserve "macho" image. Recognize

need for independence. Let choose site, etc. if
appropriate.

ADMINISTERING DRUGS

Five Rights:
>   Right drug
>   Right dose
>   Right time
>   Right route
>   Right patient

Oral medications:

Crush tablets and mix with a small amount of hot water and
then syrup. Do not mix in large volumes or add to infants bottle.
Be aware of taste. Syrups are sweet, elixirs are bitter. Use cup,
spoon, syringe, nipple (with syrups only) as appropriate for the
patient. Give slowly. If using syringe, place it halfway back at the
side of the tongue. Remember normal tongue thrust is present until
4-5 months.

Intramuscular (IM)

Sites:	Vastus Lateralis	Most meds
	Ventro Gluteal	Not until 3 years, check hospital policy
	Gluteus Maximus	Must be walking for at least 1 year, any medication.
	Deltoid	Less invasive, usually don't use until 3 years, use with non-irritating meds
Amounts:	Birth to 3 yr.	1 ml
	3-6 yr.	1.5ml
	6-15yr.	1.5-2ml
	Adult	2-3ml
Needle size:	Birth-4mo	5/8 inch
	4mo-10yr	1 inch
	10yr-Adult	1½ inch

Subcutaneous (SQ)
   Sites: Same as IM
   Amount: 0.5ml
   Needle size: 5/8-1 inch

Intravenous (IV)

Follow guidelines for proper dilution and time.
Check IV site for patency before and during infusion.
Check to be sure site and needle size adequate for volume to be
   administered. Flush IV tubing at same rate as medication
   administration to make sure all medication has been
   administered.

Rectal

Is invasive to most ages. Have preschoolers "pant like a puppy dog"
to relax sphincter. May need to hold buttocks cheeks together to
prevent expelling.

Nasogastic (NG)

Check for placement before administering meds. Be sure to flush
with water to prevent clogging tube.

Topical

Apply thin layer because of increased skin permeability.
Diaper can act as occlusive dressing and cause increased absorption
   of medication.

Eye

Put drops in inner canthus. Ointment in lower lid. Tell child that
the ointment will blur vision. If child will not cooperate, place drops
in inner canthus and hold head still so they cannot turn it to the side.
When they open their eyes to see why you haven't gone away, the
medication will go into the eye.

Ear

Less than 3 years, pull pinnae down and back to straighten ear canal. If over 3 years, pull pinnae up and back. Try to keep child on his side for one minute after administration if possible.

Nasal

Tip head back and keep back for one minute after administration of drops if possible. Remember to sit child up for administration of nasal sprays so they will properly aerosolize.

IMMUNIZATION SCHEDULE AND ADMINISTRATION

<u>Birth</u>
Hep B

<u>2 Months</u>
Hep B (May be given at 1 month)
OPV
DTP
HIB

<u>4 Months</u>
OPV
DTP
HIB

<u>6 Months</u>
OPV (High risk areas)
DTP
HIB (If using HbOC/PRP-T, not needed with PRP-OMP)

6-18 Months
Hep B (third dose must be 6 months after initial dose)

12-15 Months
MMR
HIB

15 Months
DTP or DTaP (May be given at 12 months if at least 6 months after third dose)

4-6 Years
DTP or DTaP
OPV
MMR (According to ACIP guidelines)

11-12 Years
MMR (According to AAP guidelines)

14-15 Years
Td

ACIP is the Advisory Committee on Immunization Practices
AAP is the American Academy of Pediatrics

Use IPV (Inactivated Polio Vaccine) instead of OPV when child or household member is immunocompromised, when child refuses OPV, or if initial dose is given after age 18 years.

PEDIATRIC RESUSCITATION DRUGS

ATROPINE SULFATE (anticholinergic, parasympatholytic)

Indications: Used to restore normal heart contraction during cardiac arrest. Increases heart rate and cardiac output by blocking vagal stimulation in the heart.

Administration: 0.02 mg/kg IV given slowly, minimum dose of 0.1 mg and maximum dose of 1 mg. Repeat q 5 min prn up to 1 mg for child and 2 mg for adolescent. Incompatible with sodium bicarbonate and epinephrine.

Nursing Implications: Effect on heart rate in 2 to 4 minutes. Continuous monitoring of vital signs.

BRETYLIUM TOSYLATE (antiarrhythmic)

Indications: Used in prevention and treatment of ventricular fibrillation or hemodynamically unstable ventricular tachycardia.

Administration: Unlabeled use in pediatrics. 2.5-5 mg/kg IV given rapidly over 1 minute. 10 mg/kg after 1-2 hours if necessary. Total dose not to exceed 40 mg/kg/day. Follow with continuous infusion of 1-2 mg/min or intermittent infusion of 5-10 mg/kg over 10-30 minutes q 6-8 hr.

IV dilution: Dilute 500 mg in at least 50 ml.

Compatibility: 5% Dextrose, NS, LR, 5% Sodium Bicarbonate, 20% Mannitol, Calcium Chloride in 5% Dextrose, Potassium Chloride in 5% Dextrose.

Nursing Implications: Continuous ECG monitoring needed. IV infusions should be gradually tapered. Patient is to remain recumbent to avoid postural hypotension. Usually only used if Lidocaine is not effective.

CALCIUM CHLORIDE 10% (electrolyte, calcium salt)

Indications: Used to maintain normal cardiac contractility after cardiac arrest.

Administration: 20-50 mg/kg per dose administered slowly IV. To
be repeated every 10 minutes if needed.
Compatibility: Dextrose, Sodium Chloride.
Nursing Implications: Continuous ECG monitoring needed. Patient
is to remain recumbent to avoid postural hypo-tension.

DOPAMINE (adrenergic agonist, vasopresor)

Indications: Used to treat shock and correct hemodynamics.
Improves perfusion to vital organs, increases cardiac output
and blood pressure.
Administration: 1-20 μg/kg/minute. To be increased by 1-4
μg/kg/min at 10-30 minute intervals. Dilute 200 or 400 mg in
250-500 ml of compatible solution.
Compatibility: 5% Dextrose, LR, Sodium Chloride.
Nursing Implications: Dosage is titrated to hemodynamically
desired response. Dopamine is most effective in patients who
are not hypovolemic.

EPINEPHRINE (adrenergic agonist, sympathomimetic)

Indications: Used in cardiac arrest to treat asystole. Causes
vasoconstriction, increased heart rate, and cardiac stimulation.
This is the most useful drug in cardiac arrest.
Administration: 0.01 mg/kg IV push of a 1:1000 solution. To be
repeated q 5 min prn. Intracardiac dose is 0.005-0.01 mg/kg.
Dosage should be given rapidly. Peak levels are reached 1 to
2 minutes following IV dosage.
Nursing Implications: Continuous ECG monitoring is necessary.
Drug disappears rapidly from the bloodstream. Urine formation
may decrease due to renal vessel constriction.

ISOPROTERENOL (sympathomimetic, adrenergic agonist)

Indications: Used in the management of shock and in the treatment
of cardiac standstill or arrest.

Administration: 0.1 mcg/kg/min IV initially. Increase q 5-10 min
    to desired effect up to 1.0 mcg/kg/min. Must be given diluted
    by rapid IV push. Dilute 1 to 10 ml with compatible IV solution
    for final concentration of 0.02 mg/ml.
Compatibility: Amino acids, dextrose solutions, LR, sodium
    chloride solutions.
Nursing Implications: Dosage is to be titrated to desired
    hemodynamic response. Continuous ECG monitoring is
    necessary.

LIDOCAINE (antiarrhythmic)

Indications: Used in the management of acute ventricular arrythmias
    during cardiac surgery.
Administration: Single bolus of 1 mg/kg/dose slowly IV. May
    repeat in 10-15 min x 2 (maximum dose 3.0-4.5 mg/kg/hr).
    For continuous infusion give 20-50 mcg/kg/min IV.
Compatibility: 5% Dextrose in water.
Nursing Implications: Arrange for reduced dosage in patients with
    hepatic or renal failure. Contraindicated in SA, AV, or
    intraventricular block. Prolonged infusion (24 hr) may result
    in toxic accumulation of lidocaine (therapeutic level equals
    1.5-5.0 mcg/L). Dosage is to be titrated to desired
    antiarrhythmic response.

NARCAN (narcotic antagonist)

Indications: Used to reverse the effects of narcotic depression,
    including respiratory depression induced by opioids.
Administration: Children (less than 20 kg): 0.01-0.1 mg/kg/dose
    IM/IV/SC. Repeat q 3-5 minutes as necessary. Children
    (greater than 20 kg or over 5 years): 2 mg/dose. Repeat q 3-5
    minutes as necessary.
Compatibility: normal saline, 5% dextrose in water.
Nursing Implications: Abrupt reversal of narcotic depression may
    result in nausea, vomiting, diaphoresis, tachycardia,

hypertension, and tremors. Maintain open airway and provide artificial ventilation, cardiac massage, vasopressor agents if needed to counteract acute narcotic overdosage.

NIPRIDE (antihypertensive, vasodilator)

Indications: Used for immediate reduction of blood pressure in hypertensive crises.

Administration: .5-10 mcg/kg/min. Dose titrated to a usual dose of 3-4 mcg/kg/min.

Compatibility: 5% dextrose in water.

Nursing Implications: Wrap container in aluminum foil or other opaque material to protect from light; the tubing does not have to be wrapped. Patient must be monitored with an arterial line. Do not allow BP to drop too rapidly. Provide amyl nitrate inhalation, materials to make 3% sodium nitrite solution, sodium thiosulfate on standby in case of overdose of nitroprusside - depletion of patient's body stores of sulfur occur, leading to cyanide toxicity.

PRONESTYL (antiarrhythmic)

Indications: Used to treat PVCs, ventricular tachycardia, atrial fibillation.

Administration: 20-30 mg/kg/24 hr divided q 4-6 hr IM (max dose 4 gm/24 hr). IV loading dose 2-6 mg/kg/dose over 5 min. Maintenance dose of 20-80 mcg/kg/min by continuous infusion (max dose 100 mg/dose or 2 gm/24 hr).

Compatibility: 5% dextrose in water.

Nursing Implications: Contraindicated in complete heart block. May cause lupus-like syndrome, positive Coombs', thrombocytopenia, arrhythmias, GI complaints, confusion. Monitor blood pressure and ECG when using IV. QRS widening 0.02 sec suggests toxicity. Therapeutic levels of procainamide equal 4-10 mg/L.

SODIUM BICARBONATE (electrolyte, systemic alkalinizer)

Indications: Used to treat cardiac arrest.

Administration: Infants 2 years of age: 4.2% solution IV at a rate
    not to exceed 8 mEq/kg/d; initially, 1-2 mEq/kg given over 1-2
    min followed by 1 mEq/kg every 10 min during arrest.

Nursing Implications: Monitor cardiac rhythm carefully during IV
    administration. Give slowly to prevent hypernatremia, decrease
    in CSF pressure and possible intracranial hemorrhage.

VERAPAMIL (antiarrhythmic, antihypertensive, calcium channel blocker)

Indications: Used to treat supraventricular tachyarrhythmias,
    temporarily control rapid ventricular rate in atrial flutter or
    atrial fibrillation.

Administration: For age 0-1 year: 0.1-0.2 mg/kg IV given over 2-3
    minutes. May repeat once after 30 min. For age 1-15 year:
    0.1-0.3 mg/kg IV given over 2-3 minutes. May repeat once
    after 30 min. Max dose is 5 mg.

Nursing Implications: Contraindicated in CHF, hypotension, shock,
    2nd and 3rd degree AV bock and right to left shunting. Use
    only with extreme caution in infants since it may cause apnea,
    severe bradycardia, or hypotension. Must monitor ECG
    continuously and have calcium and isoproterenol ready to
    reverse hypotension and bradycardia.

Nomogram

Place a straight edge from the patient's height in the left column to his weight in the right column. The piont of intersection on the body surface area column indicates the body surface area (BSA).

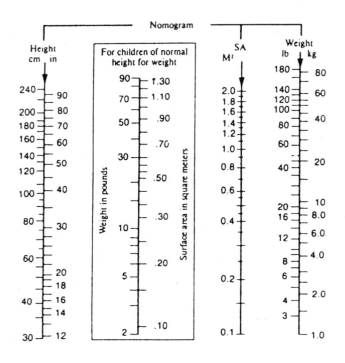

CLINICAL SKILLS

CLINICAL SKILLS
TABLE OF CONTENTS

DETERMINING ENDOTRACHEAL TUBE, LARYNGOSCOPE BLADE AND SUCTION CATHETER SIZES

AGE	WEIGHT	ETT SIZE	SUCTION CATHETER	LARYNG. BLADE
Newborn	3.0 kg	3.0-3.5	6 F	1
Infant	5.0 kg	3.5-4.0	8 F	1
1 year	10 kg	4.0-4.5	8 F	1½
3 year	15 kg	4.5-5.0	8 F	2
6 year	20 kg	5.0-5.5	10 F	2
10 year	30 kg	6.0-6.5 (cuffed)	10 F	2
Adol	50 kg	7.0-7.5 (cuffed)	10 F	3
Adult	70 kg	7.5-8.0 (cuffed)	12-14 F	3

PERFORMING CARDIOPULMONARY RESUSCITATION (CPR)

I.   Assessment

   A.   Airway patency

   B.   Assessment of respiratory status

      1.   rate - tachypnea is usually the first sign of distress

      2.   breath sounds

         a.   stridor - sign of upper airway obstruction

         b.   prolonged expiration with wheezing - sign of bronchial obstruction

         c.   diminished/absent breath sounds - sign of respiratory distress

      3.   work of breathing - respiratory effort of accessory muscle use

         a.   nasal flaring

         b.   suprasternal retractions

         c.   intercostal retractions

         d.   substernal retractions

         e.   head bobbing

         f.   see-saw respirations

      4.   color

         a.   cyanosis of mucous membranes

         b.   cyanosis of nail beds

C. Assessment of cardiovascular status

1. heart rate - infants usually respond to hypoxemis with bradycardia, whereas older children initially may be tachycardic and then bradycardic with further decompensation

2. blood pressure - hypotension is late sign

3. peripheral pulses

4. skin perfusion

   a. color

   b. skin temperature

   c. capillary refill

5. level of consciousness

6. muscle tone

7. reflex response

8. urine output - decreases as perfusion decreases (<2 ml/kg/hr in neonate; <1 ml/kg/hr in child)

II. Planning/Goal Setting

A. Obtaining equipment based upon age and size

1. resuscitation bag

2. mask - critical to achieve airtight seal

3. endotracheal tube - selection based upon child's size (cuffed tubes not necessary in children under 8)

4. laryngoscope blades - selection based upon child's age and size, straight blades preferred for neonates and infants to better visualize glottis

5. oral airway

6. suction devices

       7.   intravascular catheters

       8.   orogastric tube - to decompress air from stomach and prevent aspiration of gastric contents

  B. Maintain familiarity with equipment and location

  C. Precalculate emergency drug doses and keep at bedside

III. Implementation

  A. Determine unresponsiveness, respiratory distress, apnea, or pulselessness

  B. Call for help

  C. Position infant/child on flat, firm surface

  D. Open airway - head tilt/chin lift maneuver

  E. Observe respiratory effort

       1.   If no spontaneous respiration, begin ventilations with resuscitation bag

          a.   resuscitation bag - along with 90-100% oxygen

          b.   give two slow breaths then for

              1.   infants: 20 breaths per minute

              2.   child: 15 breaths per minute

              3.   adolescent: 12 breaths per minute

          c.   if resistance to air flow, insert oral airway

  F. For persistent resistance, suspect foreign body airway obstruction

       1.   infant

          a.   series of 4 back blows and 4 chest thrusts

       2.   child/adolescent

          a.   deliver 6 to 10 quick upward abdominal thrusts

G. Evaluate heart rate and pulses

   1. neonate - auscultate apically for 6 seconds after 15 to 30 seconds of effective ventilations

   2. infant - palpate brachial pulse

   3. child/infant - palpate carotid artery pulsations

H. Begin chest compressions

   1. neonate - digits over sternum just below nipple line, rate of 120 bpm in a ratio of 3 compressions to 1 breath, depth of 1/2 to 3/4 inch

   2. infant - fingers over sternum one finger width below nipple line, rate of 100 bpm in a ratio of 5 compressions to 1 breath, depth of 1/2 to 1 inch

   3. child - heel of hand next to index finger on sternum, rate of 80-100 bpm in a ratio of 5 compressions to 1 breath, depth of 1 to 1½ inches

   4. adolescent - heel of hand next to index finger on sternum with other hand on top locking fingers to avoid touching chest, rate of 80-100 bpm in a ratio of 15 compression to 2 breaths, depth of 1½ to 2 inches

I. Reevaluate heart rate and pulses throughout resuscitation

   1. neonate - auscultate apical pulse every 30 sec

   2. infant/child - palpate pulses after 10 cycles of compressions and breaths

   3. adolescent - palpate pulses after 4 cycles of compressions and breaths

J. Discontinue resuscitation - when heart rate is 80 bpm or greater in neonate or when pulses are palpable in infant/child/adol

K. Continue ventilations

    1. neonate - ventilate 40 times per minute until heart rate exceeds 100 bpm and spontaneous respirations present

    2. infant - ventilate 20 times per minute until spontaneous respirations present

    3. child - ventilate once every 4 sec until spontaneous respirations present

    4. adolescent - ventilate once every 5 sec until spontaneous respirations present

L. Assist with intubation if necessary

M. Obtain vascular access using large, accessible vein

N. Correctly administer emergency medications - meds used to stimulate heart rate, improve perfusion, correct acidosis, correct dysrhythmias and electrolyte imbalance

    1. central venous route (femoral, internal/external jugular, subclavian and umbilical veins) -more rapid onset and higher peak concentration

    2. peripheral venous (scalp, cephalic, basilic, antecubital, saphenous, and dorsal arch of hand or foot)

    3. intraosseous (tibia in infants/young children) - used to infuse fluids, epinephrine, whole blood, calcium, lidocaine, atropine, and sodium bicarb

    4. endotracheal tube - used to administer certain meds when vascular access not available

O. Insert orogastric or nasogastric tube -helps to prevent aspiration

P. Correct other problems during resuscitation

    1. acidosis

    2. hypoxemia

    3.   hypothermia

    4.   hypocalcemia/hypoglycemia

IV. Evaluation Outcomes

  A. Resuscitation occurs promptly

  B. Child is adequately oxygenated/ventilated

  C. Child is well perfused

  D. Child experiences minimal or no complications

V. Documentation

  A. Events preceding the arrest

  B. Time and type of arrest

  C. Interventions performed

  D. Personnel involved

  E. Child's response to interventions

  F. Time when resuscitation efforts stopped

ISOLATION PROCEDURES AND UNIVERSAL PRECAUTIONS

I.   Body substance isolation or Universal Precautions: Major difference is the BSI system considers all patients potentially infectious for all pathogens while UP system considers all patients potentially infectious and requires additional protection once diagnosis is made. Most institutions have adopted one of these two systems recommended by the Center for Disease Control.

II.   Body substances considered potentially infectious

    A. BSI - all including blood, feces, urine, vomitus, wound and other drainage, oral secretions

    B. UP - blood, semen, vaginal secretions, CSF, synovial fluid, pleural fluid, peritoneal fluid, pericardial fluid, amniotic fluid. Fluids not included UNLESS they contain blood: feces, nasal secretions, sputum, sweat, tears, urine, vomitus

III. Handwashing

    A. BSI - performed for 10 sec with soap, running water, and friction any time the hands are visibly soiled and between patient contact even if gloves worn

    B. UP - Immediately and thoroughly wash hands and other skin surfaces that are contaminated with body fluids to which UP apply

IV.   Protective gloves

    A. BSI - must be worn when contact with mucous membranes, nonintact skin, or moist body substances is likely to occur. Must be changed in between patients.

    B. UP - must be worn when touching fluids to which UP apply

V.   Gowns

    A.   BSI - should be worn when it is likely that body substances will soil clothing. Should be changed in between patient contacts.

    B.   UP - same as with BSI

VI. Masks/eye protection

    A.   BSI - should be worn when likely that eyes and/or nose and mouth will be splashed with body substances or when working over large, open skin areas

    B.   UP - same as with BSI

VII. Sharp disposal

    A.   BSI - should not remove needles from disposable syringes. Needles should not be recapped. Sharps and needles to be disposed in puncture resistant container in close proximity to patient contact

    B.   UP - same as with BSI

VIII.Trash and linen disposal

    A.   BSI - bagged in leak proof container

    B.   UP - same as with BSI

IX. Private rooms

    A.   BSI - a private room is desirable for children who soil environment with body substances. It is required for children with airborne, communicable disease unless roommate shown to be immune to the disease.

    B.   UP - not addressed other than to use disease or category specific isolation precautions. Diseases that require the use of strict or respiratory isolation include varicella, diphtheria, mumps, pertussis, measles, erythema infectiosum, epiglottitis, meningitis, pneumonia.

SPECIMEN COLLECTION

Urine Collection

Infants—Clean area and allow to dry. Prepare area with Benzoin if skin is intact, let dry until its sticky and attach pedi urine bag. Can extract urine from bag with a small gage needle and leave bag attached if still need more urine. Young infants have a reflex that if they are suspended supine on nurses hand, she can press at base of spine and gently stroke upward with two fingers. This causes infant to arch back, raise buttocks in the air, cry, and void if their bladder is full. Allows for quick collection of specimen in bag or cup held under the infant.

Toddlers—place hat type specimen collection container in the hole in their potty chair. Then they can void normally and not have to "perform" by voiding in a cup.

Stool Collection

If need to collect loose stool in infants to send for electrolytes, can bag the anus using a pedi urine bag.

Blood Collection

Warm extremity before capillary draws. Wipe area with alcohol again after the stick to increase blood flow. Squeezing the extremity or digit can increase hemolysis and artificially elevate potassium results. Capillary Hct can be 5-10% higher than venous Hct. For venous collections, the antecubital vein is best for all age groups and hurts less than using veins on the hand or foot.

TIPS

To Encourage Fluids

Melt popsicles in microwave until slushy. Child can then eat it with a spoon or straw. Feels good on sore throats.

Offer a 5-10cc syringe. Show child how to draw up liquid and squirt it in their mouth. Works best with 3-10 year olds. Improves intake because its fun.

To Encourage Deep Breathing

Have child blow bubbles or a pin wheel. Can have them "blow out the light" with a pen light. Have them blow a cotton ball across the bedside table into a paper cup and pretend its a soccer or hockey goal.

To Decrease Gagging

Gently press back on the chin to help stop gag reflex. Works best in young infants.

Fussy Babies

If have assured baby is not hungry or needs changing, check to be sure the IV has not infiltrated. This is the most common cause of continued fussy baby's. Expose IV as much as necessary to ensure patency. Compare extremities for size and shape to determine swelling.

If IV is patent, try rocking motions, soothing voice, singing or music to calm baby.

IV Starts in Infants

Best site for young infants is the head. It causes less restrictions in movement and the least amount of disturbance in achievement of developmental tasks. Infants forget it is there and leave it alone. If infiltrates, causes less tissue damage because circulation to area is less impaired than in the extremities. When use the scalp, save a lock of the infant's hair that is shaved for the mom to put in the baby book to remember first "hair cut". This helps ease mom's chagrin over the infant having their head shaved.

Warm Soaks

Warm soaks to extremities stay warm longer if the extremity is wrapped in a warm wash cloth and then "diapered" with a disposable diaper. The plastic helps keep the warmth in longer and keeps the bed from getting wet.

DISEASE PROCESSES AND COMMON PROBLEMS

DISEASE PROCESSES AND COMMON PROBLEMS

TABLE OF CONTENTS

SEIZURES

DESCRIPTION

Abnormal electrical discharges from the brain which cause paroxysmal, uncontrolled episodes of behavior. The consequences of this activity can include: (1) alteration in responsiveness, (2) alteration in sensation/perception, and/or (3) alteration in movement/mobility/muscle tone.

PATHOPHYSIOLOGY

Pathophysiology of seizures is unclear. Causes range from acute central nervous system disorders (i.e., hypoxia, infection, head injury, toxin exposure, tumors, fever) to idiopathic, unknown factors.

DIAGNOSTIC TESTS

CT Scan, MRI, EEG, skull radiography, EMG, brain scan, lumbar puncture, antiepileptic drug blood levels.

NURSING ASSESSMENT

Need to distinguish seizures from breath holding spells, hyperventilation, postural hypotension, mitral valve prolapse, hypoglycemia, tourette syndrome, sleep disorders. Prompt recognition of seizure activity is necessary. Careful seizure observation and documentation is necessary. Describe the beginning of the episode including any precipitating factors. Describe the patient's response to self, nurse, and environment. Assess response to auditory, tactile, and visual stimuli. Describe movements, mobility, and tone. Observe exact location including whether one side of the body or both sides are affected. Assess whether muscle tone is increased or decreased. Assess sensation and perception by asking child to describe what is happening. Assess child for any postictal responses. Note how long it takes for child to resume previous activities.

NURSING CARE

Stay with child during seizure. Protect child from potential injury (i.e., falls, aspiration pneumonia, hyperthermia, drug side effects). Be sure not to restrain child's movements. Reorient child after episode while providing reassurance and psychosocial support for child and family. Emergency assistance should be sought if (1) respiratory arrest, (2) seizure activity lasts for greater than 5 minutes (status epilepticus), (3) multiple seizure episodes occur without return of consciousness in between (status epilepticus), and/or (4) the child has sustained injury.

IV or rectal administration of antiepileptic drugs such as diazepam, phenytoin, and phenobarbital is done during episodes of status epilepticus. Knowledge deficit is a common patient problem. The nurse is involved with instructions related to seizures, antiepileptic drugs, diagnostic tests, seizure recognition, and first aid.

INSULIN DEPENDENT DIABETES MELLITUS

DESCRIPTION

IDDM is the most common endocrine disorder of childhood. IDDM is referred to as Type I diabetes. There is an absolute deficiency of pancreatic insulin. The result is chronic high blood sugar and other problems with carbohydrate and fat metabolism. The mode of inheritance is still not well-described. There is some evidence that genetic predisposition is an important factor. Viral infection is thought to be a significant antecedent. The disease is characterized by polyuria, polydipsia, polyphagia, and fatigue. Weight loss prior to initial diagnosis is also common.

DIAGNOSTIC TESTS

Glucose tolerance test, HbA1c (to assess long term metabolic control), blood glucose monitoring, urine testing for ketones.

PATHOPHYSIOLOGY

Inadequate secretion of insulin results in decreased glucose transport from the bloodstream into the cells which leads to hyperglycemia. Triglycerides are metabolized into free fatty acids. These are converted into ketoacids by the liver and are used for energy. Glucagon is secreted and leads to production of glucose from glycogen and from amino acids which further raises blood glucose.

NURSING CARE

For diabetic ketoacidosis (DKA): Assess vital signs, q 15 min initially then q 1 hr until stable. IV fluid replacement involves initial administration of NS then D5.45NS when blood sugar < 300. Assess hydration. Administer insulin (usually given IV when child is dehydrated). Hourly blood glucose & electrolyte levels are drawn. Cardiac monitoring used to detect arrhythmias related to potassium imbalance.

After DKA resolves need to teach safe administration of insulin, teach about insulin type, dosage, and mixing of insulin. The child and/or parent is taught about injection sites and the protocol for rotating sites. Dietary management is taught which includes consistent meal times, no concentrated sweets, and specified meal plan. The nurse also plays and important role in facilitating the child and family's adjustment to diabetes. Strategies to improve self-care management are discussed.

ASTHMA (REACTIVE AIRWAY DISEASE)

DESCRIPTION

Chronic pulmonary disease which results from a wide range of stimuli (i.e., pollen, dust, virus). Results in increased irritability of tracheobronchial tree with airway obstruction of varying degrees. The condition is usually reversible following therapy or spontaneously. Children are more vulnerable to airway obstruction because of their small airway and compromised collateral ventilation.

PATHOPHYSIOLOGY

Narrowing of airway is caused by (a) smooth muscle contraction of the airway, (b) edema of the tracheobronchial mucosa, and (c) excessive secretion of submucosal glands which causes mucous plugging.

DIAGNOSTIC TESTS

CBC (leukocytosis occasionally found, eosinophilia frequently found), serum IgE, PFT's, peak expiratory flow rate, chest radiograph, skin testing for allergies.

NURSING ASSESSMENT

Obtain thorough history. Children with asthma frequently have history of eczema, recurrent bronchitis, persistent coughing. Symptoms usually are worse at night. Respiratory assessment should include respiratory rate, presence of dyspnea, retractions, nasal flaring, and the use of accessory muscles. Skin color and capillary refill time should be noted. Lungs should be auscultated for unequal breath sounds, crackles, and/or wheezing. Cardiac rate and rhythm should be assessed especially during drug therapy.

NURSING CARE

Provide patient teaching related to avoidance of allergens and or triggers. Administer drug therapy. Theophylline may be used IV during severe episodes. Adrenergic drugs such as albuterol may be used po or by aerosol. Cromolyn is used as a preventative medication. Glucocorticosteroids may be given by inhaler, po, or IV. Provide oxygen and place in Fowler's or semi-Fowler's position. Arterial blood gases are obtained. Provide teaching related to home care. Often children are discharged on inhaled medications and/or steroids.

RESPIRATORY SYNCYTIAL VIRUS (RSV)

Infective Organism:

Respiratory Syncytial Virus. Type A is more virulent than Type B.

Sources:

Humans

Transmission:

Predominantly through direct contact with respiratory secretions mainly by hand to eye, nose, or other mucous membranes. Airborne transmission has not been documented.

Incubation period:

Usually 5-8 days

Signs and symptoms:

The signs and symptoms are more pronounced in young infants. Illness usually begins with a upper respiratory infection. Rhinorrhea and fever appear first. Conjunctivitis and otitis media are commonly seen with RSV. As the disease progresses it becomes a lower respiratory tract infection. Classic symptoms include wheezing, retractions, crackles, dyspnea, tachypnea, and diminished breath sounds.

Isolation:

Strict contact isolation and handwashing. Gowns may be used to help diminish potential spread of the organism. The number of hospital personnel, visitors, and uninfected patients in contact with the child should be diminished during acute outbreaks.

Nursing care:

High humidity and adequate fluid intake should be provided. Often mist therapy is combined with oxygen by hood or tent in order to alleviate dyspnea and hypoxia. IV fluids may be preferred during the crisis of the disease in order to conserve energy needed for oral feedings. Close respiratory assessment, oxygen saturation monitoring, and blood gas analysis are used to guide therapy. Bronchodilators, steroids, antibiotics, and cough suppressants have not proved to be effective in the treatment of RSV. An antiviral agent, Ribavirin, is the only specific therapy available for RSV. The medication is delivered via a small-particle aerosol generator (SPAG). The use of this agent is restricted to those children with underlying medical conditions which place them at a high risk for complications. The drug is teratogenic. Health care personnel and visitors who might be pregnant should avoid contact with the child during Ribavirin therapy.

Complications:

Potential for respiratory compromise.

COMMUNICABLE DISEASES

CHICKEN POX (VARICELLA)

Infective Organism:

Varicella-zoster virus (Herpesvirus)

Sources:

Humans

Transmission:

Direct contact with respiratory secretions, also airborne

Incubation period:

Usually 14-16 days

Signs and symptoms:

Very pruritic rash begins on the trunk as macules and progresses to vesicles and crusting. May have slight fever and decreased appetite.

Isolation:

Strict isolation for 5 days minimum after rash begins and until no new lesions formed and all vesicular lesions are crusted.

Nursing care:

Symptomatic. No aspirin. Acetaminophen may delay crusting. Tepid bath with corn starch may help with itching. Administer Benadryl or Atarax as ordered for itching. Keep child's nails short. Teach older child to push on itching lesions instead of scratching. Keep child cool to decrease itching and lesion formation.

Complications:

Local cellulitis from secondary infections. Encephalitis. Reyes syndrome.

MEASLES (RUBEOLA)

Infective organism:

RNA virus

Sources:

Humans

Transmission:

Direct contact with droplets, less commonly airborne

Incubation period:

Usually 8-12 days

Signs and symptoms:

Fever, cough, coryza, conjunctivitis with photophobia, Koplik spots on the posterior buccal mucosa, followed in 2-3 days with an erythematous maculopapular rash beginning on the face and spreading downward. Rash is confluent and turns brownish in color after 3-4 days. Skin may peel over heavily rashed areas.

Isolation:

Respiratory isolation for 4-5 days after onset of rash.

Immunocompromised children need to be isolated for the entire course of illness because of prolonged excretion of the virus in respiratory secretions.

Nursing care:

Symptomatic. Bedrest, antipyretics, dim lights, cool mist vaporizer, tepid baths

Complications:

Otitis media, pneumonia, encephalitis, and rarely subacute sclerosing panencephalitis (SSPE)

MUMPS

Infective organism:

Paramyxovirus

Sources:

Humans

Transmission:

Direct contact with respiratory secretions

Incubation period:

Usually 16-18 days

Signs and symptoms:

Fever, headache, malaise, followed by swelling and pain of one or both parotid glands

Isolation:

Respiratory isolation until 9 days after onset of parotid swelling.

Nursing care:

Supportive. Bedrest, antipyretics, analgesics, increase fluids, soft bland diet, hot or cold compresses to parotid glands.

Complications:

Encephalitis, orchitis.

RUBELLA (GERMAN MEASLES, 3-DAY MEASLES)

Infective organism:

RNA virus

Sources:

Humans

Transmission:

Direct or droplet contact with nasal secretions. Infants with congenital rubella shed the virus in nasopharyngeal secretions and urine up to one year or more.

Incubation period:

14-21 days, but usually 16-18 days.

Signs and symptoms:

Postnatal: pinkish-red maculopapular discrete rash beginning on the face and progressing rapidly downward and covers the body the first day. Disappears in the order it came usually by day three. Accompanied in older children by low grade fever and generalized lymphadenopathy, especially suboccipital, cervical, and post-auricular. Transient polyarthralgia and polyarthritis common in adolescent girls.

Isolation:

Postnatal: contact isolation for the first 7 days after onset of rash. Congenital: consider contagious until one year old.

Nursing care:

Supportive. Antipyretics for fever and analgesics for discomfort.

Complications:

Encephalitis, thrombocytopenia — rare. Biggest complication is the teratogenic effect on the fetus.

PERTUSSIS (WHOOPING COUGH)

Infective organism:

Bordetella Pertussis

Sources:

Humans

Transmission:

Close contact via respiratory secretions.

Incubation period:

6-20 days, usually 7-10 days

Signs and symptoms:

Mild upper respiratory symptoms progressing to severe paroxysms of coughing with an inspiratory "whoop" followed usually by vomiting. Fever, if present is usually low grade.

Isolation:

Respiratory for 5 days after beginning Erythromycin or until three weeks after onset of cough if not treated with Erythromycin.

Nursing care:

Administer Erythromycin as ordered, otherwise supportive with bedrest until no fever, encourage fluids, and increase humidity via humidifier or tent. Refeed after vomiting. Observe for airway obstruction.

Complications:

Pneumonia, seizures, hernia, prolapsed rectum, encephalopathy, death.

TUBERCULOSIS (TB)

Infective organism:

Mycobacterium Tuberculosis

Sources:

Humans. Children usually get it from infected adults

Transmission:

Inhalation from infected respiratory droplets from an adult with infectious pulmonary TB.

Incubation period:

From infection to TB skin test being positive is 2-10 weeks. Risk for developing disease state is greatest in the first 2 years after infection but can be many years later. Most become dormant.

Signs and symptoms:

Positive Mantoux test using 5 tuberculin units of purified protein derivative (PPD) administered intradermally indicates infection. Positivity interpreted as follows as recommended by the American Academy of Pediatrics Committee on Infectious Diseases. These recommendations apply regardless of BCG administration.

Reaction ≥ 5mm

—children in close contact with persons with known or suspected infectious TB

—children suspected to have TB because of a positive chest x-ray or clinical evidence of TB

—children with immunosuppressive conditions including immunosuppressive dose of corticosteroids or HIV infection

Reaction ≥ 10mm

—children at increased risk of acquiring TB due to:

Young age (less than 4 years old)

Medical risk factors of Hodgkin's lymphoma, Diabetes Mellitus, chronic renal failure, malnutrition

—children with increased environmental exposure:

Foreign born or children of parents born in regions of increased TB incidence

Frequent exposure to adults who are HIV positive, homeless, drug users, poor and medically indigent city-dwellers, residents of nursing homes, institutions or prisons, or migrant farm workers

Reaction ≥ 15mm

—children ≥ 4 years old without any risk factors

Most children are asymptomatic. Early manifestations include lymphadenopathy, pulmonary involvement with or without consolidation, pleural effusion, miliary TB and TB meningitis.

Isolation:

Most hospitalized children need no isolation if they are receiving drug treatment. Those with positive AFB in sputum smears should have respiratory and contact isolation until after treatment effective and sputum shows decreasing organisms and cough is going away.

Nursing care:

Appropriate testing and interpretation. Isolation if necessary. Administer medication as indicated and education of parents of the importance of compliance with preventive chemotherapy. Preventive chemotherapy usually is with INH 10mg/kg/day for 9 months given QD. (Max 300mg). Those with active disease are treated with 6, 9, or 12 month regimes depending on the site of infection using a combination of 2,3,or 4 of the following drugs: Isoniazid, Rifampin, Pyrazinamide, or Streptomycin. Partial treatment can lead to drug resistance. All children with active TB should have HIV testing. Ensure nutritious meals, adequate rest and monitor growth and development.

Complications:

Drug resistance, adverse reactions to drug therapy.

<u>HIV INFECTION</u>

Infective organism:

Human immunodeficiency virus type 1

Sources:

Humans

Transmission:

Predominant modes are from sexual contact, exposure to contaminated needles or other sharp instruments, or mother to infant transmission before or around the time of birth.

Incubation period:

Variable from months to years. Perinatally infected median age of onset is age 3 years. Those who acquire it other than perinatally usually develop serum antibodies to HIV within 6-12 weeks after infection.

Signs and symptoms:

Can present in any system. Most common manifestations include generalized lymphadenopathy, hepato and splenomegaly, failure to thrive, recurrent or persistent oral candidiasis and recurrent diarrhea. Also may show developmental delay, lymphoid interstitial pneumonitis (LIP), recurrent invasive bacterial infections, and opportunistic infections such as pneumocystis carinii pneumonia (PCP).

Diagnostic testing:

HIV ELISA—enzyme-linked immunosorbent assay for HIV antibody. Is a screening test.

HIV Western Blot—confirmatory test used to check the validity of the ELISA test because it more precisely detects the presence of antibodies to specific antigens.

HIV p24 Antigen Assay—tests for a protein that surrounds the RNA and reverse transcriptase of the HIV

HIV PCR—a polymerase chain reaction.

HIV Culture—this with the HIV PCR are the most sensitive and specific tests to determine HIV infection in children who were perinatally exposed.

Classification:

As of 1994 (MMWR, 1994), children with HIV infection are classified by 3 immunologic and 3 clinical categories:

Immunologic categories

Categorizes by the severity of immunosuppression caused by the HIV infection. Age specific CD4 counts and T-lymphocyte percentages determine the category.

1. No evidence of suppression

2. Evidence of moderate suppression

3. Severe suppression

Clinical categories

Used to provide a staging classification.

N. Not symptomatic

A. Mildly symptomatic

B. Moderately symptomatic

C. Severely symptomatic

The best prognosis is a child classified as N1. Poorest would be C3. Specific parameters and definitions have been established by the CDC. E prefix means perinatally exposed.

Isolation:

Universal blood and body fluid precautions.

Nursing care:

Depends somewhat on the child's classification and condition. Many have multiple hospitalizations and need the same care as other children with chronic or life-threatening illnesses. Need to help support the family and child emotionally by listening and helping set up services as needed. Utilize social services and all resources available in the community. Growth and development surveillance is important. Protect from secondary infections with good handwashing and protective isolation as warranted by their CD4 and T-lymphocyte counts. Help keep hydrated, maintain good nutrition and encourage development as much as tolerated. Administer antibiotics and antifungals as ordered. Education on the transmission and prevention of HIV infection.

Complications:

Failure to thrive or HIV wasting syndrome, loss of developmental milestones, multiple and persistent infections, LIP (lymphoid interstitial pneumonitis), PCP (Pneumocistis carinii pneumonia), HIV encephalopathy, death.

CONGENITAL CARDIAC DEFECTS AND REPAIRS

Presenting signs and symptoms:

History

Poor feeding, decreased weight gain, tires with feeding, sweating, frequent respiratory infections, breathes fast or hard, can't keep up with peers, tires easily

Physical exam

Tachycardia, bradycardia, tachypnea, elevated BP, palpable thrills, decreased pulses, poor perfusion, murmurs

Work-up:

Chest x-ray (CXR)—to determine heart size and location
Electrocardiogram (EKG)—to measure electrical activity of the heart

Holter monitor—24 hour monitoring of heart rate and rhythm

Echocardiogram (ECHO)—sound waves show images of heart formations

Cardiac catheterization—catheter is advanced usually through the femoral vessels to visualize heart structures and blood flow patterns and measure pressures and oxygen levels

Common defects and repairs:

Defects causing an increase in pulmonary blood flow

ASD (Atrial Septal Defect)—an opening between the atriums. Usually repaired with a patch closure.

VSD (Ventricular Septal Defect)—an opening between the ventricles. Small ones repaired with a pursestring suture, large ones with a patch.

AV Canal (Endocardial Cushion Defect)—a low ASD continuous with a high VSD and cleft of the mitral and tricuspid valves. Palliative treatment is to do a pulmonary artery banding (PA Banding). Full repair involves patch closure of the septal defects and reconstruction of the valve tissue. Some need mitral valve replacements.

PDA (Patent Ductus Arteriosus)—when the fetal ductus does not close. Can be treated by surgical ligation, with a clip closure, or is sometimes occluded during cath.

Obstructive defects

COA (Coarctation of the Aorta)—narrowing of the aorta at the insertion of the ductus arteriosus. Surgical repair involves resection with end to end anastomosis or enlargement of with a graft.

AS (Aortic Stenosis)—narrowing or stricture of the aortic valve, can lead to hypertrophy of the left ventricle. Treated surgically with aortic valvotomy or valve replacement. Sometimes can dilate narrowed valve with a balloon angioplasty in the cath lab.

PS (Pulmonary Stenosis)—narrowing of the entrance to the pulmonary artery, can lead to right ventricular hypertrophy. Pulmonary Atresia-is a fused valve that allows no blood flow to the lungs and can cause a hypoplastic right ventricle. Treated with a transventricular valvotomy (Brock Procedure) or a balloon angioplasty in cath lab.

Defects causing a decrease in pulmonary blood flow

TOF (Tetralogy of Fallot)—consists of 4 major problems: VSD, PS, overriding aorta, and right ventricular hypertrophy. Palliative treatment with Blalock-Taussig (BT) shunt or modified BT shunt to provide pulmonary blood flow from right or left subclavian arteries. Complete repair is preferred and involves closure of the VSD, resection of the stenosis, and a pericardial patch.

Tricuspid Atresia—failure of the tricuspid valve to develop. Palliative treatment is placement of a pulmonary to systemic shunt to increase the blood flow to the lungs and a second stage of a bidirectional Glenn shunt. Repair is done with a modified Fontan procedure.

Mixed defects:

TGA (Transposition of the Great Arteries)—pulmonary artery arises from the left ventricle and the aorta from the right so there is no communication between the systemic and pulmonary circulation. Is incompatible with life without associated mixing defects such as a PDA, ASD, or VSD. Palliative treatment with prostaglandin to keep the PDA open, and balloon atrial septostomy (Rashkind procedure). Surgical repair with arterial switch within the first weeks of life. Senning procedure with an intraatrial baffle using the atrial septum, Mustard procedure using prosthetic material can be done with older children. A Rastelli procedure is used when the child has TGA, VSD, and severe PS.

TAPVC (Total Anomalous Pulmonary Venous Connection)—the pulmonary veins don't join the left atrium. Surgical treatment varies with the anatomical defect.

Truncus Arteriosus—the pulmonary artery and the aorta didn't separate and override both ventricles. Treated with a modified Rastelli procedure.

HLHS (Hypoplastic Left Heart Syndrome)—underdevelopment of the left side of the heart leading to a hypoplastic left ventricle and aortic atresia. Surgical treatment with a multiple stage Norwood procedure or a heart transplant in the newborn period.

Nursing care:

<u>Preop:</u>

Assess vital signs, exercise tolerance, provide adequate nutrition, rest. May need to space care to conserve child's energy. Maintain hydration. Assess for signs and symptoms of congestive heart failure (CHF): Tachycardia, diaphoresis, decreased perfusion, cold extremities, mottling, duskiness, tachypnea over 60, retractions, cyanosis, orthopnea, cough, wheezing, failure to thrive, hepatomegaly, edema, and/or abnormal weight gain. Assess development. Teach parents how to care for child at home or to prepare for surgery if imminent. Provide comfort, administer diuretics, cardiac meds as ordered. Neutral temperature of environment conserves energy. If post cath, observe for bleeding and assess circulation of involved extremity.

<u>Postop:</u>

Assess vital signs. Provide for rest, comfort (administer pain meds as ordered) encourage fluids, progressive ambulation, and emotional support. Observe for the following complications:

Infection—fever, foul smelling drainage, increased pain
CHF—Signs and symptoms described above
Cardiac tamponade—narrowing pulse pressure, tachycardia, dyspnea, cyanosis, apprehension, tripod position.

Heart Block—usually bradycardia
PPS (Post Pericardial Syndrome)—fever, chest pain, irritability
Prepare for discharge by teaching parent how to care for child at home and encourage normalcy.

CARE OF CHILDREN WITH CHRONIC DISEASES

The number of children with chronic diseases and conditions are increasing. These children and their families have unique responses, needs and nursing care requirements.

Affect on child

Unpredictability can lead to frequent hospitalizations and doctors appointments that interrupt normalcy. May have associated pain, discomfort. Child may have misinformation or not enough information and fear the unknown. Their growth and development may be restricted and this makes them different from their peers. They may be unable to participate in normal activities and this also makes them feel different from their peers. May have decreased feelings of worth and feel guilty for daily care requirements.

Child's response

The child may respond by being angry, uncooperative, and belligerent. May show signs of depression, resignation or confusion. They may also feel isolated and withdraw.

Affect on family

Grieve for the loss of the normal child and their potential. Feel a strain on all relationships. Stress over daily care requirements and financial burden. May feel loss of control and isolation.

Parent's response

The type of chronic illness and amount of positive feedback from the child affect the parent's response. Parents may go through denial, grief, guilt, anger, helplessness, fear and loneliness. These feelings may be potentiated at every missed milestone such as first steps, first day at school, getting a driver's license, etc.

Sibling's response

May feel forgotten, less important and jealous of sick sibling. They may get angry and resent the parents being away all the time. They may feel guilty, sad, isolated, or lonely, and may act out to get attention.

<u>Nursing Intervention</u>

General

Utilize primary nurse as much as possible, and admit to same unit in the hospital. Use a developmental approach instead of one based on age to help emphasize abilities and not disabilities. Focus on strengths. Encourage normalcy as much as is realistic. As families learn their child and their condition, they become the experts for that child and need to be recognized as such.

Child

Depends on age and condition. Assess the child's understanding of their illness and how they are responding and adapting. Provide support for coping and allow and encourage expression of feelings. Promote normal growth and development. Prepare for changes and treatments. Encourage participation in care and control and responsibility for as much as possible. Encourage peer support and help with care. Help them to understand expectations and responsibilities. Focus on abilities. Encourage association with peers with the same problems if possible and encourage involvement in decision-making.

Parents

Assess where the parents are in adapting to the child's illness. Determine and provide the knowledge, skills or resources needed to help them adapt. Encourage involvement of both parents. Clarify needs of each parent. They may be in different stages of adapting due to amount of contact with the child and the health care system. Encourage normalization and realistic expectations of the child and family functioning. Encourage open communication. Allow verbalization of frustrations and feelings, and respond in a caring, nonjudgmental, nondefensive manner. Help them to get involved in parent support groups if appropriate and to set up their own support systems.

Siblings

Encourage visitation and involvement in care during hospitalization if appropriate for siblings age and child's condition. Assess their understanding of the child's illness and their adjustment to it. Provide supportive communication. Encourage phone calls to the parents and sick child. Give positive strokes when present and recognize their presence and feelings.

DEALING WITH DYING

Death is a difficult nursing situation because it causes nurses to examine their feelings about death, their own and others. Working with dying children and their families can be both challenging and rewarding. To be most effective, nurses need to be aware of how different age groups conceptualize and react to death, their own and others.

Perceptions by Age Groups

Infants/Toddlers
Concept: None.

Rxn to Own Impending: Take questions from loved ones responses.
Rxn to Death of Others: React to the separation and loss of consistency by regressing, becoming irritable, and have sleeping and eating problems.

Preschoolers (3-5 years)

Concept: It is separation, temporary, gradual, and reversible.
Rxn to Own Impending: It is a punishment for bad thoughts or actions.
Rxn to Death of Others: They may feel guilty, as if their thoughts or actions were responsible. May regress or show denial with inappropriate behavior.

Schoolagers (6-9 or 10 years)

Concept: It is not reversible but also is not inevitable. May personify it. May see it as destructive or look for natural or physical explanations.
Rxn to Own Impending: May show fear of the unknown. Need help to maintain control of own body. May be verbally uncooperative due to fear. Show "flight or fight" reaction.
Rxn to Death of Others: Feel guilt and responsibility. Ask many questions to help them arrange facts into concrete and logical understanding.

Adolescent (9 or 10 years to adult)

Concept: It is irreversible, universal and inevitable. It is a personal but far off event. They explain it physiologically and theologically.
Rxn to Own Impending: They reject death because it interferes with their establishment of identity. Become alienated from their peers and unable to talk to parents. Use denial and rationalization. Are present oriented and worry about physical changes that may further alienate them from their peers.
Rxn to Death of Others: Feel guilt and shame. Have the most difficulty coping with death of all the age groups.

Parent Responses

Initial (When informed of life threatening illness or   condition of the child)
Shock, disbelief
Anger
Become overprotective
Anxious
Ambivalent

After the Loss
Shock, confusion, decreased sense of reality
Guilt, anger
Sorrow
Depression
Loneliness, yearning
Helplessness, despair, fear
Reorganization, reconciliation, relief

Both parents may be in different stages of acceptance and respond totally differently. The parents may have reached acceptance before the nurse does. They may be reconciled to the death of their child long before the child dies. They need to be helped to understand and not feel guilty for their feelings.

Sibling Responses

Siblings respond according to their age group and developmental stage. Their reaction also is dependent on the parental reaction, the amount of time they have had to adjust and the amount of involvement and inclusion they have had. They often feel isolated and guilty. They may also feel that they are not as important as the child who died, that they need to replace that child and be strong, be good, and not talk about their sibling. They may have been sheltered and left out.

Nursing Care of the Dying Child and Their Family

Nurses may need help in dealing with their own feelings before they are able to help the dying child and his family. Seek assistance from experienced nurses, the social worker or chaplain. Every nurse is initially uncomfortable because it forces us to face our own mortality. Be careful to not impose your own views, values, or explanations on the family.

Child

The dying child needs accurate, honest information and time to think it out. There needs to be a gradual process with increasingly open communication between the child, the parents, and the nurse. When the child asks questions, ask them what they think is happening to see what they understand, how they feel and what they really want to know. Be sure to discuss with the parents before as to how they want to handle communication and what they want the child to know. Even though open communication is best, it is still the parent's right to determine what they feel is best for their child. Help correct any misinformation.

Family

Assess their ability to cope and resources and intervene or refer as necessary. Parents also need honest and complete information to empower them to make appropriate choices. They need information on how to tell the child, siblings and other family members. They need an opportunity to express their feelings in a supportive environment. Respect their wishes in regard to what they want the child to know, but help them to realize that trust fosters trust. After the death of the child, stay with the family or have a chaplain or social worker available. Ensure the child's dignity. Encourage expression of memories, feelings. Answer questions honestly. Allow them to stay with the child as long as they wish. Give them time and privacy to say goodbye. Help with arrangements, ensure closure, encourage ties.

CLINICAL REFERRALS

CLINICAL REFERRALS
TABLE OF CONTENTS

RESOURCES FOR CHILD-HEALTH NURSING AND 1-800 NUMBERS

GENERAL CHILD HEALTH

Aid to Adoption of Special Kids   (800)232-2751

American Academy of Pediatrics   (800)433-9016
    141 Northeast Point Blvd.
    P.O. Box 927
    Elk Grove Village, IL 60009-0927

Healthy Mothers, Healthy Babies Coalition   (800)673-8444
    Match parents of children with special needs
    MUMS—Mothers United for Moral
        Support, Inc.   (414)336-5333
        150 Custer Court
        Green Bay, WI 54301
    NPPSIS—National Parent to Parent Support and
        Information System   (800)651-1151
        P.O. Box 907
        Blue Ridge, GA 30513

National Center for Education in Maternal &   (202)625-8400
    Child Health

AIDS/HIV

National AIDS Hotline   English   (800)342-2437
                          Spanish   (800)344-7432

National Pediatric HIV Resource Center   (800)362-0071

ASTHMA

Asthma & Allergy Foundation of America   (800)7-ASTHMA
    1125 15th ST., NW, Suite 502   (202)466-7643
    Washington, D.C. 20005

National Heart, Lung, & Blood Institute
    National Asthma Education Program   (301)251-1222
    NIH Building 31, Room 4A21
    9000 Rockville Pike
    Bethesda, MD 20892

BIRTH DEFECTS/CRIPPLED CHILDREN

Association of Birth Defects in Children   (407)859-2821
    3526 Emerywood Lane
    Orlando, FL 32812

Blind Children's Center   (800)222-3566

Deafness Research Foundation   (800)535-3323

Infant's With Disabilities & Life-Threatening
    Conditions National Clearing House   (800)922-1107

March of Dimes Birth Defects Foundation   (914)428-7100
    1275 Mamaroneck Ave.
    White Plains, NY 10605

National Down Syndrome Society   (800)221-4602

National Easter Seals Society for Crippled
    Children   (800)221-6827
    70 E Lake St.
    Chicago, IL 60612

United Cerebral Palsy Association   (800)872-1827

CANCER

American Cancer Society   (800)ACS-2345

The Candlelighters Childhood Cancer Foundation (800)366-2223
    7910 Woodmont Ave, Ste. 460
    Bethesda, MD 20814

The Leukemia Society of America, Inc.   (800)955-4572
    600 Third Ave
    New York, NY 10016

National Cancer Institute   (800)4-CANCER
    NIH Building 31, Boom 10A24
    9000 Rockville Pike
    Bethesda, MD 20892

DIABETES/RENAL

Juvenile Diabetes Foundation   (800)JDF-CURE

National Kidney Foundation   (800)622-9010

DIET

American Dietetic Association   (312)899-0040
    216 W. Jackson Blvd.
    Chicago, Ill. 60606

Mead Johnson Nutritionals   (812)429-5000
    2400 W. Lloyd Expressway
    Evansville, IN 47721

National Dairy Council   (708)696-1020
    6300 N. River Rd.
    Rosement, IL 60018-4233

DRUG ABUSE

800 Cocaine   (800)262-2463

Drug Abuse Hotline   (800)662-HELP

National Clearing House for Alcohol & Drug
    Information   (800)729-6686

National Council on Alcohol & Drug Abuse   (800)622-2255

National Institute of Drug Abuse   (800)729-6686

National Parents' Resource Institute for
    Drug Education   (800)667-7433

HEART DISEASE

American Heart Association   (800)242-8721
    National Center
    7320 Greenville Ave.
    Dallas, TX 75231

MENTAL HEALTH

National Autism Hotline   (800)525-8014
National Mental Health Association   (800)969-6642

OTHERS

American Burn Association   (800)548-2876
Cleft Palate Foundation   (800)242-5338
Cystic Fibrosis Foundation   (800)FIGHTCF
Epilepsy Information Service   (800)642-0500
National Association for Sickle Cell Disease (800)421-8453
National Attention Deficit Disorder Association (800)487-2282
National Council on Child Abuse and Family
    Violence   (800)222-2000
National Head Injury Foundation   (800)444-NHIF
National Hemophilia Foundation   (800)42-HANDI
National Organization of Rare Disorders   (800)999-6673
Neurofibromatosis Foundation   (800)323-7939
SIDS Alliance   (800)221-SIDS
SIDS National Headquarters   (800)222-SIDS

PEDIATRIC NURSING JOURNALS

JOURNAL OF PEDIATRIC HEALTH CARE

National Association of Pediatric Nurse Associates and
Practitioners
Mosby-Year Book Inc.
11830 Westline Industrial Dr.
St. Louis, MO 63146-3318

JOURNAL OF PEDIATRIC NURSING

Nursing Care of Children and Families
W.B. Saunders Company
6277 Sea Harbor Dr.
Orlando, FL 32887-4800

MATERNAL/CHILD NURSING

The American Journal of Maternal/Child Nursing
Box 53435
Boulder, CO 80322-3435

PEDIATRIC BASICS

Medical Services Dept., Gerber Products Co.
Fremont, MI 49413

PEDIATRIC NURSING

A. Jannetti Publications, Inc.
East Holly Avenue Box 56
Pitman, NJ 08071-0056

REFERENCES

American Nurses' Association. (1983). <u>Standards of Maternal and Child Health Nursing Practice.</u> Washington, DC.

Center for Disease Control and Prevention: 1994 Revised classification system for human immunodeficiency virus infection in children less than thirteen years of age. <u>MMWR</u> 43: 1-10, 1994 (No. RR-12).

Committee on Infectious Diseases. (1994). <u>Report of the committee on infectious diseases.</u> (23rd ed.) Elk Grove Village: American Academy of Pediatrics.

Deglin, J.H. & Vallerand, A.H. (1996). <u>Davis's drug guide for nurses</u>. (4th ed.) Philadelphia: F.A. Davis

Frankenburg, W.K. & Dodds, J.B. (1990). Denver II. Denver: Denver Developmental Materials, Inc.

Fuller & Schaller-Ayes. (1994). <u>Health Assessment.</u> (2nd ed.) Philadelphia: J.B. Lippincott.

Hazinski, M.F. <u>Nursing Care of the Critically Ill Child.</u> St. Louis: Mosby Year Book.

Johnson, K.B. (1993). <u>The John Hopkins Hospital, The Harriet Lane Handbook.</u> (13th ed.) St. Louis: Mosby Year Book.

Pillitteri, A. (1995). <u>Maternal & Child Health Nursing.</u> St. Louis: CV Mosby.

Wong, D.L. (1995). <u>Waley and Wong's Nursing care of infants and children.</u> (5th ed.) St. Louis: Mosby Year Book.

Wong and Whaley. (1990). <u>Clinical Manual of Pediatric Nursing</u>, St. Louis: Mosby Year Book.

INDEX